Patsy Westcott is one of *Mother & Baby* magazine's top journalists.

CW01072742

By the same author

Pregnancy and Birth
Your Baby's First Year
Your Child's Health

The
Mother & Baby
Book of

FEEDING YOUR
BABY AND CHILD

Patsy Westcott

GRAFTON BOOKS
A Division of the Collins Publishing Group

LONDON GLASGOW
TORONTO SYDNEY AUCKLAND

Grafton Books
A Division of the Collins Publishing Group
8 Grafton Street, London W1X 3LA

A Grafton Paperback Original 1990

A CIP catalogue record for this book is available from the British Library

ISBN 0-586-20664-7

Printed and bound in Great Britain by
Collins, Glasgow

Set in Goudy Old Style

CONTENTS

INTRODUCTION

Parents, and mothers in particular, often become aware of food in a whole new way when they have a baby to feed. But while supermarkets now contain a greater variety of produce than ever before, food can be a headache for today's parents. Scarcely anyone can be unaware of the links that have been made in recent years between diet and health. But how can parents decide what to put on the weekly menu when today's goodies become the baddies of the food world overnight? Just what is a healthy diet? And how can you ensure that your child eats one?

We at *Mother & Baby* are used to these sorts of questions. In this book we aim to provide clear, sensible guidelines for feeding your child from birth to three years. In the first chapter we discuss feeding your new baby. We look at the benefits of breast-feeding, and how you can get feeding off to a good start. If you cannot manage or do not want to breast-feed, bottle-feeding is a safe alternative. We offer advice on how you can bottle-feed happily and tips for successful feeding from the early days to the last bottle-feed.

Chapter two looks at the question of introducing solids. New mothers often worry a great deal about when and how to start. This chapter tells you all you need to know, from how to tell when your baby is ready for solids, to food preparation tips and a suggested weaning schedule.

Chapter three takes you on to the toddler years. It looks at what food your child should eat, how to plan a menu, and how to deal with the common problem of a faddy eater.

Chapter four contains food facts designed to help you plan your child's menu so that it provides maximum nourishment.

The next chapter concerns your child's growth. It sets out average rates of growth so you can compare your child, looks at problems such as overweight, and offers useful tips on what you can do about them.

Many more parents nowadays are vegetarian, and chapter six deals with the nutritional needs of the vegetarian baby and toddler. It will be especially useful to those vegetarians who have not been brought up vegetarian themselves, and will do much to reassure such parents that they can give their child a healthy, nourishing diet without meat.

There has recently been an increase in the number of allergies reported, yet a good deal of confusion surrounds the subject, and also that of artificial additives in our food. In an effort to set the record straight, chapter seven deals with these two related subjects. It tells you all you need to know about food additives, and offers useful tips on how to deal with food allergy or intolerance.

Chapter eight is for parents whose children have special dietary needs. It sets out the feeding requirements of premature babies so you can ensure your premature baby gets all the necessary nutrients. There is information for the mother who wants to breast-feed her premature baby. Babies and toddlers are often hardest to feed when they are ill, so we also look at ways in which you can cater for your child at these times. Finally we look at special diets for two of the most common medical conditions requiring one – diabetes and coeliac disease – and emphasize that though your child may need to select food carefully there is no need to feel different from other children.

Last but not least we have included a range of simple, easy-to-prepare recipes designed for busy mothers – for babies from six months who are just starting solids, to family meals suitable for older babies and toddlers. This section also includes a wide range of vegetarian recipes, healthy puddings and suggestions for teatime treats that are bound to appeal to toddlers.

We hope this book helps you to provide your child with a diet that will ensure strong and healthy growth, as well as taking the worry out of eating so that you and your child can discover that food is fun.

Patsy Westcott, 1990.

Note: In order to reflect the experiences of all mothers, 'he' and 'she' have been alternated chapter by chapter in this book to refer to the child.

1 EARLY DAYS

In the first few weeks at home with your baby you will find that most of your time seems to be spent feeding. You need to decide in advance which method of feeding will suit you, your baby and your lifestyle best.

Babies thrive on milk, either from the breast or a specially modified formula for the first few months. You can combine breast- and bottle-feeding if this fits in with your life better.

Although breast milk has never been rivalled as a food for babies, modern formulas enable bottle-fed babies to thrive quite happily. When deciding how you will feed, do bear in mind that feeding involves more than simply meeting your baby's nutritional needs. Some women feel distaste for the whole idea of breast-feeding. Others find having total responsibility for a tiny baby overwhelming, and may feel they need the space and freedom offered by giving a bottle. Some women – although only a very small minority – cannot breast-feed for medical reasons affecting either themselves or their babies.

This section offers information to help you make up your mind, tips on how to feed your baby, whichever method you choose, and answers some of the questions that new mothers ask. You will also find detailed information on both breast- and bottle-feeding in *The Mother & Baby Book of Pregnancy and Birth* and *The Mother & Baby Book of Your Baby's First Year*. Happy feeding!

BREAST-FEEDING – OFF TO A GOOD START

There is no doubt that, if you can manage it, breast is best for your baby. Breast milk is so perfectly adapted to the needs of the human baby that no formula milk, however cleverly modified, matches up to it. Breast-feeding not only has health benefits for your baby now, but these benefits are thought to continue into later life, long after you have stopped breast-feeding.

Breast-feeding takes a little while to establish, so do persevere if you have problems. Once any initial difficulties are overcome most mothers find breast-feeding quick, easy and convenient. It helps to know a little about how breast-feeding works, and ways in which you can overcome any early problems.

WHY BREAST-FEED?

- Human milk is the perfect food for babies. It contains exactly the right balance of nutrients for your baby, and this adjusts automatically to cater for your baby's changing needs.
- Breast-fed babies suffer fewer infections, especially gastroenteritis, which is especially dangerous to young babies. This is because breast milk contains special substances that actively protect your baby from infection.
- Breast-fed babies suffer fewer allergies. Research suggests that babies who are exposed to 'foreign' proteins such as cow's milk can develop an allergic reaction, which may persist into childhood. Complete breast-feeding for six months may protect your baby from developing allergies if there is a family history of them.
- Breast-feeding confers long-term health benefits. People who were breast-fed as babies are said to be less at risk from heart disease, certain digestive disorders, and tooth decay.
- Breast-feeding gives your baby instant comfort, automatically providing the physical closeness that babies need.
- Breast-fed babies seldom get constipated – and their nappies smell sweeter!
- The changing composition of breast milk during a feed helps develop appetite control – one reason why breast-fed babies are less likely to grow up to be overweight.
- Breast-feeding is cheaper. You do not have to buy bottles, teats, sterilizers and packets of milk.
- Breast-feeding is more convenient. The milk is always there, at the right temperature and in the right quantities for your baby, whenever and wherever he wants feeding.
- Breast-feeding is best for you: it helps your womb shrink back to normal size, and it delays the return of your periods – a plus point for those who have had difficult periods before childbirth.
- Breast-feeding helps you lose weight by using up stores of fat laid down during pregnancy. Some women, however, do not regain their usual figure until after they have stopped feeding.
- Breast-feeding is pleasant for both you and your baby. Nothing can

compare with the satisfaction of seeing your baby grow and knowing it is all your own work. Mothers who breast-feed often comment on the special closeness they feel for their baby.

HOW TO ENJOY BREAST-FEEDING

You will enjoy breast-feeding more if you are armed with a few simple facts about breast-feeding, and one or two practical tips.

During pregnancy. Find out about the breast-feeding policy at your local hospital. You will need lots of support and encouragement from those around you in the early weeks, when there may be one or two minor difficulties to overcome. Find out whether you will be encouraged to put your baby to the breast immediately after delivery – so long as he is fit and well. An early start to breast-feeding helps. Ask if feeding is encouraged 'on demand' – that is, where you pick up your baby and feed him whenever he appears to be hungry. Are you allowed to keep your baby with you at all times – this is known as rooming-in? Or if your baby is taken to the nursery, for instance when you are tired, will the staff bring him to you for feeding when he wakes? Ask how many mothers leave hospital fully breast-feeding their babies – if the answer is seven out of ten, or higher, you can be sure that mothers are receiving the help and support they need. Some hospitals have a special lactation or breast-feeding sister to help new mothers become happily established with feeding. Certainly this cuts down on unhelpful conflicting advice and information, which can be so confusing in the early days.

Discuss your wish to breast-feed with the sister at the antenatal clinic. She will examine your breasts to make sure they are suitable for breast-feeding. An important consideration is your nipples. Do they stand out when you are cold, when you handle them, or when you are sexually excited? If they remain flat or turn inwards – that is, if they are 'inverted' – you may need a little extra patience and perseverance in the early days of breast-feeding. This is not a major problem, and once you have had your baby his sucking will usually be sufficient to draw out your nipples. However, there are one or two things you might like to try during pregnancy which could help. You can obtain some special plastic 'shells' to wear inside your bra during pregnancy, which will help gently draw out your nipples. These are available on prescription. Ask your doctor or midwife if you think you would like to try them. In addition you (or your husband) can gently roll your nipples between thumb and forefinger to encourage them to protrude. Use a lanolin cream or baby oil to make this easier.

If you do not have inverted nipples there is no need to do anything special to prepare for breast-feeding. A daily bath or shower is enough to keep your breasts clean, but go easy on the soap, as it can dry up the natural oils that keep your nipples supple. You can massage a little cream into your breasts after bathing, but it is not essential. In summer try going topless if you can find a spot that isn't overlooked – the sun and air will help prepare your skin for breast-feeding, but do use a high-protection-factor sunscreen.

You will need to buy two or three well-fitting bras. The sort that double as nursing bras after the baby is born are the best value. Choose cotton or cotton mix, and look for wide straps and good support beneath the breasts and at the sides. The bra should fit snugly with no gaping, but it should not be tight.

Research has shown that mothers who breast-feed are the ones who have been breast-fed themselves, and whose husbands support their decision to breast-feed. Your own views and your attitude towards your body and its functions also have a part to play. These will have been shaped by what you have seen and read, the experiences of friends and relatives and, if you have other children, whether or not you breast-fed them and enjoyed it.

It is worth considering these questions and trying to sort out your feelings about breast-feeding before you have your baby. If you are undecided, it is worth trying to breast-feed. You can always swap to the bottle if you find breast-feeding does not suit you. Even though it is possible to change from bottle to breast it is easier the other way round, and just a few days of breast-feeding will give your baby an excellent start in life.

If breast-feeding does go badly at first, try not to give up too easily. Most breast-feeding mothers report that it takes a good six weeks for their milk supply to adjust to the baby's demands, and the less you interfere with this natural process (for example by giving additional bottles) the sooner you will settle down to happy breast-feeding.

Most mothers who give up in the early weeks do so because they fear that they are not producing enough milk. It is all too easy to believe this when faced with a fretful baby and no visible means of seeing how much milk your baby is getting. However, breast-feeding works by a system of supply and demand and the best way to boost your milk supply is to be patient and to put your baby to the breast as frequently as possible.

HOW YOUR BODY MAKES MILK

One of the first signs of pregnancy is an increase in the size of your breasts. This is caused by the growth of milk-producing cells and ducts, which during pregnancy and during the time you are breast-feeding replace the fatty padding in your breasts. It is not necessary to have big breasts in order to breast-feed. Women with small breasts manage just as well.

During pregnancy hormones from the placenta and your pituitary gland trigger off production of the special early milk, colostrum. You may notice crusts of this, or a slight leakage of yellowish fluid from your nipples, after about the fifth month of pregnancy.

The really dramatic changes occur after your baby is born. From about the third or fourth day after birth, hormonal changes sparked off by birth and by your baby suckling set in motion milk production. Before that, your breasts produce a special high-protein fluid called colostrum which also has anti-infective properties. During this start-up period your breasts will feel heavy and full (engorged). Rest assured that this uncomfortable stage usually passes off within a day or so.

Your breasts will remain fuller than usual for the first month or so of breast-feeding, and then they usually return to their normal pre-pregnancy size. This is not a sign that you are producing less milk, simply that the right balance has been struck between your supply and your baby's demands.

THE VITAL 'LET-DOWN'

Breast-milk production is governed by hormones that are released by the stimulation of your baby's sucking. That is why *the more often you let your baby suck at your breasts the more milk will be produced.* The milk is produced deep inside your breast and flows down through ducts and out in several jets through the nipple as a result of what is called the 'let-down reflex'. This is a muscular reflex sparked off by hormones, which causes the milk to be squeezed through the milk ducts and into the small sacs that lie deep under the areola (the dark ring around the nipple). The baby squeezes on these sacs with his gums as he sucks. The let-down reflex is extremely sensitive. It can be triggered off by thinking about your baby or hearing him or another baby crying. It can also be held back if you are tired, tense or in pain. In this case, although your baby will get some milk, it will be the low-fat 'foremilk'. The more satisfying 'hindmilk', which contains more calories and so ensures he feels satisfied, remains in the breast. One of the main reasons some mothers do not produce enough milk in the early days is that the let-down reflex has failed to work – either for the reasons mentioned above, or because your baby is not properly on the nipple.

How do you know whether you are getting a 'let-down'? One sign is a tingling, sometimes almost painful sensation in the nipple, a few seconds or minutes after the baby has been put to the breast. Another is when milk starts to drip from the breast at which the baby is not feeding, shortly after the feed starts. The hormones involved in the let-down are the same ones that cause your uterus to contract during labour, and mothers of second or subsequent babies often experience 'afterpains' in the abdomen as the uterus shrinks down in the first week or so after birth.

BREAST MILK – NATURE'S WONDER FOOD

There have been many attempts to create a formula that meets all a baby's needs in exactly the same way as breast milk does. However, although today's modified baby milks are as close to human milk as is technologically possible, none so far matches breast milk. For a start, breast milk varies from one mother to another, and from day to day. The type of milk produced by the mother of a pre-term baby differs from the milk of mothers of full-term babies. The volume and composition of your milk is unique to you and your baby. It alters throughout each day according to your sleeping and eating patterns. Breast milk contains cells, enzymes and special proteins that carry antibodies and protect your baby against many infectious illnesses.

Colostrum is the earliest form of milk to be produced during pregnancy. Your baby needs only a small amount of this highly concentrated fluid, which is specially designed for the newborn baby, but it is very precious. Colostrum provides all the nutrients, including water, that your baby needs in the first few days after birth. It is high in protein and vitamins A and B12, but lower in fat than mature breast

How to ensure you have a good let-down

- Feed your baby whenever he seems hungry.
- Do not limit the time your baby sucks at the breast.
- Make sure your baby is on the breast properly. His mouth should be well sealed around the areola, and there should be no gap between his chin and your breast. You should also notice the little muscles at the sides of his ears working as he sucks!
- Try to relax. Make yourself comfortable, and have a drink handy, as breast-feeding may make you thirsty. Practise slow, calm breathing. Play some soothing music. If you feel embarrassed about feeding in front of others, find a quiet corner to feed in.
- If your baby's sucking does not appear to be triggering the reflex, try bathing your breasts in warm water before a feed.
- If you are having severe let-down problems, ask the midwife or doctor if they advise using a special hormone nasal spray which triggers off the let-down reflex.
- Get plenty of rest and relaxation, and remove obvious sources of stress and worry.

milk. Above all, colostrum is rich in antibodies, which line the baby's gut and block harmful bacteria and viruses. Because colostrum is so rich, your baby will sleep a lot in the first few days after birth. It also has a laxative action which helps to clear out your baby's intestinal system.

Gradually, between about the third to the tenth day after birth, colostrum begins to give way to mature breast milk. By comparison with colostrum, which is thick and creamy in appearance, breast milk looks thin, bluish and watery. This is how it is meant to look. It doesn't mean it is too weak or thin for your baby. Breast milk contains all the ingredients your baby needs in exactly the right quantities to facilitate strong and healthy growth. Despite continuing research, formula makers still do not yet know all the constituents of breast milk. So long as you are in reasonable health and are eating a good diet, breast milk will contain all the vitamins, major minerals and trace elements your baby needs, in a form which he can easily absorb. Human milk contains less protein than cow's milk because babies grow more slowly than young calves.

Breast milk contains a type of milk sugar called lactose, which is thought to aid the absorption of calcium and balance the bacterial levels in the gut. The fat content of breast milk is higher than that of formula milks, and provides your baby with energy. It also carries vitamins that dissolve in fat, such as vitamins A, D, E and K, and vital prostaglandins – special hormone-like substances responsible for regulating many bodily functions. The fat in breast milk is different from that found in artificial milks. It is used more efficiently by your baby's body and contains a type of fat that helps absorption. It is thought that this type of fat is important in the growth of the brain and the nervous system. Moreover, the fat content of milk changes during the course of a feed: at first the baby takes in low-fat, thirst-quenching

Five tips for easy breast-feeding

- *Put your baby to the breast as soon as possible after birth.* The sucking reflex is strongest in the period immediately after birth. Surveys have shown that frequent early feeding helps get breast-feeding well established. If you cannot feed your baby straight away because one of you is ill, don't be anxious. If your baby has to spend some time in special care being tube fed, ask the staff if you can keep up your milk supply by expressing or pumping off milk with a hand or electric pump (see pages 94–5).
- *Feed your baby whenever he seems hungry.* Frequent suckling increases your milk supply and reduces the risk of painful engorgement. Your baby may want to be fed as often as every two hours in the early days. Bear with this, and by the end of the first week his demands will become less frequent. As the weeks go by, the length of time between feeds will gradually increase.
- *Feed your baby from both breasts.* This ensures that both breasts are equally stimulated. In practice your baby will usually empty the first breast and drink as much as he likes from the second. Start the next feed on this second breast to ensure even emptying. A small safety pin fastened to your bra strap on the appropriate side will help you remember which side to start on. If your baby occasionally falls asleep after just one breast, it doesn't matter. The chances are he will wake a little earlier for his next feed, and you can give him the other breast first.
- *Avoid complementary bottles and other drinks.* Breast-feeding works on a system of supply and demand. Breast milk alone contains all your baby needs, including water. If you give your baby complementary bottles (extra drinks of baby milk in addition to his breast-feed) perhaps because of uncertainty, or because you are afraid he is not getting enough, your breasts will not receive enough stimulation to produce the amount of milk your baby needs. Another result of giving complementary feeds is that your baby may discover that it is easier to suck from a bottle, and he will be less inclined to suck at the breast. This in turn reduces the amount of stimulation your breasts receive.
- *Do not overdo it.* Your flow of milk is affected by psychological and physical factors such as worry, tiredness and so on. Find a quiet place to feed, then relax and enjoy it.

'foremilk' but, as he continues to feed, richer milk is released from deep inside the breast by the let-down reflex. The fat content of this is three to four times higher than that of foremilk, and provides your baby with a feeling of fullness and satisfaction.

GETTING STARTED – HALF THE BATTLE

You can put your baby to your breast as soon as he is breathing well, or crying, and has had any mucus sucked out of his air passages. This first feed will soothe and comfort him after the stress and strain of being born. Of course, if your baby is unwell or needs medical attention, you may have to delay this feed. In this case breast-feeding may take a little longer to establish, so don't despair; patience and perseverance will win the day.

Don't worry if your baby doesn't learn to suck properly straight away. With time and practice he will soon be an expert. If you have had drugs such as pethidine too close to the birth, or if your baby has had a difficult birth, he may be drowsy and uninterested in feeding to start off with. Again, perseverance will do the trick.

Positioning. Getting your baby into a good position for feeding is important – not only so that he can give your nipples the right amount of stimulation to produce milk but also to avoid sore nipples. The main cause of sore nipples is that the baby is chewing on the end of the nipple rather than pressing against the sacs which lie beneath the areola. Make sure that your clothes are not preventing him getting close enough. Ask your midwife to help you put your baby on the breast. Don't rush it; if your baby is not keen to suck, let him nuzzle and lick your nipple and try again a little later. He won't starve if he doesn't get the knack of feeding straight away.

QUESTIONS AND ANSWERS ABOUT BREAST-FEEDING

Q. *My baby starts to suck and promptly falls asleep. Is there anything I can do?*
A. There may be several reasons why your baby is sleepy and uninterested in feeding. It could be that drugs you were given during labour are still circulating in his system. Or perhaps you are taking other medicines such as sleeping pills. Pain-relieving drugs will

gradually pass out of your baby's system and he will become more alert. If you are taking sleeping tablets, are you sure they are really necessary? Try deep breathing, relaxation, or listening to a soothing tape before bedtime. A warm bath and a drink of herbal tea such as chamomile will also help soothe and relax you. Hospitals are often kept at sub-tropical temperatures, with the result that a baby may be drowsy. Try unwrapping your baby to cool him down, and hold him in a fairly upright position to discourage him from falling asleep. If he won't feed, try again a little later. Take advantage of any alert spells to feed him. If it is very hot in your room, try opening a window.

Some babies get jaundiced after birth, which makes them sleepy. The jaundice is harmless and passes off with time. It is caused by a build-up of bile products in the blood, due to your baby's immature liver. Feeding often helps flush the jaundice away. In severe cases your baby may need to be placed under a special light panel (phototherapy) to help clear the jaundice. Once your baby has recovered he will be a more lively feeder.

It could be that your baby is not grasping the nipple correctly. If he just nibbles on the end his sucking reflex will not be triggered, he won't get much milk, and may become discouraged and uninterested. Make sure he is well on to the breast. Ask the midwife to help you settle into a comfortable position.

Aim for at least six feeds a day. Your baby may need several more, especially during the first two weeks.

Q. *My baby seems hungry all the time. Is he getting enough?*
A. It is quite normal for a breast-fed baby to want feeding often – as frequently as two hourly – in the early days. This is nature's way of ensuring that your milk supply increases to meet his needs, and will also help prevent any uncomfortable build-up of milk in your breasts (engorgement). Most babies lose a little weight at first and it can take up to three weeks before they gain it again.

It is natural to worry that your baby is not getting enough. But so long as your baby has plenty of wet nappies, has yellow, soft bowel motions and seems alert and responsive, the chances are he is fine. Having your baby weighed regularly should help reassure you that he is thriving.

Signs of underfeeding are dry nappies, scanty, dry, greenish bowel motions, no weight gain, or weight loss (after the first few days). The remedy is to feed more often to boost your supply. Breast-feeding will always soothe a fretful baby.

Try to get rest and relaxation yourself and eat well. Avoid giving complementary bottles as they will reduce your supply.

Babies undergo frequent leaps in growth (growth spurts). These often happen around the 10th to 14th day after birth, and again at three weeks, six weeks, and three months. Extra feeding will usually create a bigger milk supply and your baby will become more settled.

If your baby is not gaining weight, problems with your let-down could be the cause. Relax before feeding, and check that the baby is on the breast properly.

When you first arrive home with your baby his demands may seem overwhelming. Try to gain a sense of perspective by keeping a diary of your baby's feeding and sleeping times. It is normal for your baby to feed six to eight times a day, and he would do this even if he were bottle-fed. You may find a sort of pattern emerging when you check his feeding and sleeping habits over the course of a few days. Use this to plan your own time for yourself.

Q. *My baby never seems to settle, and I'm at the end of my tether. Could it be my milk?*
A. Breast milk is perfectly suited to your baby, so your milk is unlikely to be the cause. Although breast milk looks thin and watery it contains all the nutrients your baby needs. Your baby may be hungry (see above), in which case you should increase the number of feeds you give. Eat well and relax. But he may simply be bored and want some company. After the first couple of weeks many babies do not sleep very much. Try carrying him in a sling, or placing his bouncing chair where he can see you. Talk to him and recognize him as the individual he is.

Your baby could even be too full, or windy. Encourage him to burp by holding him upright against your shoulder. Some babies with very rapid weight gain suck a lot for comfort. You could try encouraging a longer gap between feeds, by delaying the start of a feed next time he wakes up, or distracting him by playing with him, giving him a bath, or taking him out in the pram.

If your baby seems to be crying all the time, keep a crying diary. You may be surprised to find it is not as much as you think. Plan distractions for times when he is crying. Swaddling, warmth, rocking can all help. Alternatively try a baby-soothing cassette. These are available from

Ameda Baby Ssh, Ameda Ltd, Unit 2 Belvedere Trading Estate, Taunton, Somerset TA1 1BH; Jaygee Cassettes, 19 Golf Links Road, Burnham-on-Sea, Somerset TA8 2PW; Dawne Baby Shusha, Dawne Instruments Ltd, 4 Donkin Road, Armstrong Industrial Estate, Washington, Tyne and Wear NE37 1PF.

If you are reaching the end of your tether, contact your health visitor. For help and support write to Crysis, BCM Cry-sis, London WC1N 3XX.

Q. *I'm fully breast-feeding my baby. What shall I do when I want to go out?*
A. There are two options here. Firstly, you can take your baby with you. If you think you would feel embarrassed about feeding in front of other people, experiment with shawls and big, baggy sweatshirts or T-shirts before you go out. You'll find that with a little imagination it is perfectly possible to feed so discreetly that only you and the baby know what you are doing!

Secondly, you can leave the baby with his father or a babysitter with a bottle of milk in case he gets hungry. This could be either a bottle of expressed breast milk, or a modified baby milk. Once breast-feeding is established it is superbly flexible. You can collect breast milk by wearing plastic shells to collect the drips that come from the other breast while you are feeding, and storing the milk in a sterilized bottle in the fridge. Expressed breast milk will keep for six months in the freezer, and 24–48 hours in the ordinary part of the fridge. Alternatively you can express with a pump or by hand. You can do this after a feed if the baby hasn't fully emptied one breast or, if your baby has dropped a night feed, before you go to bed.

Q. *Can I still breast-feed if I return to work?*
A. Many mothers have successfully combined breast-feeding with working. If you go back to work while your baby is still having several feeds a day, you will need to do a bit of juggling. You can either leave bottles of expressed breast milk to be given to your baby in your absence, or alternatively combine breast- and bottle-feeding. You can arrange his routine so that you give him a breast-feed immediately before leaving for work and as soon as you get home. Depending on your working hours and whether you are full or part time, whoever is looking after your baby may need to give only one or two feeds while you are away.

It is probably a good idea to get your baby used to sucking from a bottle at an early age, so that he does not reject the unfamiliar feel of the teat when you return to work. You can get him accustomed to this by bottle-feeding him expressed breast milk once or twice a week once he is a few weeks old.

If you are planning to give your baby expressed breast milk while you work, then as soon as you get home from hospital start collecting your milk and storing it in the freezer after feeding and if there is any to spare. You may need to express using a hand or electric pump while you are at work. This will only be practical if there is a quiet place where you can do this.

Of course, if you are not planning to return until seven months or so after your baby's birth, your baby will be eating some solids by then and your milk supply will have diminished accordingly.

For more advice and hints on happy breast-feeding, see *The Mother & Baby Book of Pregnancy and Birth* and *The Mother & Baby Book of Your Baby's First Year.*

For further tips on combining breast-feeding and working, contact one of the following breast-feeding organizations:

Association of Breast-feeding Mothers, 18 Lucas Court, Winchfield Road, London SE26 5TJ. Tel: 01-778 4769.
La Leche League BM 3424, London WCIV 3XX. Tel: 01-242 1278.
National Childbirth Trust (Breast-feeding Promotion Group), Alexandra House, Oldham Terrace, London W3 6NH.
Tel: 01-992 8637

BOTTLE-FEEDING – HOW TO SUCCEED

Breast may be best for babies, but one in five mothers does not manage to breast-feed, and many others change to bottle-feeding after a period of breast-feeding. It is reassuring to know that modern infant formulas are more sophisticated and closer to breast milk than ever before. So long as you follow a few simple hygiene rules bottle-feeding is completely safe, and countless babies thrive on it perfectly happily. It is also possible to give your bottle-fed baby the same love and closeness that you would if you were breast-feeding.

WHY BOTTLE-FEED?

The overwhelming advantages of breast-feeding are for the baby, but in the case of bottle-feeding the advantages are mainly for the parents. However, as more relaxed parents generally make for a happier baby you should not feel guilty or worry that you are depriving your baby by opting for or switching over to the bottle.

The biggest bonus of bottle-feeding is that the baby is not entirely dependent on you for feeds. If you are planning to return to work soon after your baby is born, or if you lead a very active social life, then bottle-feeding may well fit in better with your lifestyle.

Bottle-feeding also allows the baby's father to play a bigger part in child care during the early months. Another advantage mentioned by some women is that you can see exactly how much milk the baby is getting. If you are the type of person who finds the sight of those ounces going down reassuring then bottle-feeding may suit you better.

Some new mothers find the responsibility of caring for a new baby awesome. If you feel like this, bottle-feeding may well be better for you because it distances you slightly and allows you to share the responsibility and take some time off.

WHICH MILK?

Ordinary cow's milk is unsuitable for babies under one year old. Unmodified cow's milk has much higher concentrations of minerals than breast milk, making it unsuitable for a baby's kidneys to cope with. It also contains types of fat and protein that are not easily digestible.

At present there are about 10 different brands of modified baby milks on the market. These conform to strict DHSS guidelines, and their composition has been carefully worked out so that they are as close as possible to breast milk.

There is slightly more protein in modified baby milks than in breast milk. This is to compensate for the fact that it is slightly less well absorbed than the protein found in breast milk. Levels of carbohydrate are raised to make them more similar to breast milk, and some of the naturally occurring fats are replaced with blends of fat that come closer to those in human milk. Mineral and vitamin levels are adjusted until they are similar to those found in human milk. All modified baby milks are fortified with vitamin D and with iron, which is less readily absorbed from cow's milk.

There are no clear advantages of one brand over another, but mothers and professionals often have their own personal preferences. The main difference between the brands is in the type of protein found in them. Whey-based formulas are said to resemble human milk more closely than those that have a higher proportion of casein (milk curds). The protein in them derives from the whey part of cow's milk, which is easily digested by babies. Because casein stays in the baby's stomach for longer, it is often claimed that such milks are more satisfying for the baby. However, the difference is marginal.

In curd-based formulas the protein content derives from the casein, or curd part of cow's milk. This takes longer for the body to process so it may be more suitable for older babies or for those who appear hungrier.

There is another group of artificial feeds based on non-milk protein (usually soya). These have been developed for babies who are allergic to cow's milk or who have special needs because of prematurity or illness. You should use these brands only on the advice of your doctor.

From the age of six months or so, breast and bottle-fed babies can be given follow-on formula, which is a modified cow's milk with added vitamins and minerals.

Try not to make the mistake of thinking that a satisfied baby is one who sleeps for four hours between feeds. Breast-fed babies usually want feeding much more often than every four hours. Four-hourly routines are based on the days when baby milks were less like breast milk and had to be given at fixed intervals to ensure the baby did not put too great a strain on his system by having too much milk. Modern modified milks can be fed on demand just like breast milk. After the first few weeks healthy babies are alert and aware between feeds, and enjoy being with the rest of the family.

You will find more details about the composition of artificial milks in *The Mother & Baby Book of Your Baby's First Year*.

Baby milks are available either ready made or as powders or liquids to which you add water. The ready-made version, which is probably what you will use in hospital, is more expensive to buy.

MAKING UP BOTTLES

Always follow the manufacturer's instructions to the letter. If you do change brands check the instructions, and use the scoop provided. Never add extra formula to the bottle, as this concentrates the feed and can overload your baby's kidneys.

You may find it more convenient to make up a 24-hour supply of your baby's feeds in advance and store it in the fridge. Alternatively you can make up each bottle as you need it. At first the instructions for making up and sterilizing may seem daunting, but with practice you will soon become an expert.

1. Choose a time of day when you will not be interrupted: early morning, or before you go to bed are generally convenient.
2. Check the kitchen to make sure it is clean and free from flies, and shut out any pets. Wash the kitchen table, or whichever surface you plan to use for preparation.
3. Wash your hands well and dry them on a clean towel.
4. Get together all the equipment and a kettle of freshly boiled water that has been slightly cooled. Do not use water that has been boiled more than once or water that has gone through a water softener, as the mineral content may have been concentrated and could put a strain on your baby's kidneys.
5. Rinse the bottles with boiled water then pour the correct amount of boiled water into the bottles and, using the scoop provided, measure out the stated amount of milk powder. Be careful not to pack the scoop too full or to compress the powder, or you could end up with a too-concentrated feed. Level the power by scraping the top of the scoop lightly with the back of a knife. Always add the powder to the water and not the other way round.
6. Fit the teats and bottle caps and shake gently until the feed is well mixed. You may prefer simply to fit the bottle caps and leave the teats in sterilizing solution until feed time.

WARMING UP BOTTLES

Don't give your baby his bottle straight from the fridge as it might chill him. Some babies will take their bottle at room temperature but many find it more comforting if it is warmed. Either stand the bottle in a basin or jug of hot water, or use an electric bottle warmer. Do not warm up milk in a microwave once you have put it in the bottle, as the fluid in the middle of the bottle may become very hot and scald the baby.

Always test the temperature of the feed on your wrist before giving it to the baby.

Don't let the feed stand about in a bottle warmer, as this can breed germs. As soon as it has reached the correct temperature, feed it to your baby.

At night, or if you are away from home, you need to think ahead. A bottle will keep for a couple of hours once it has been taken from the fridge, but if you need to keep it for longer you should store it in a clean, insulated cool-bag until you need it. You can keep a bottle warmer beside the bed, or take it out with you. Alternatively take a thermos flask full of hot water in which to stand the bottle. Never keep milk warm in a flask as this forms an ideal breeding ground for harmful bacteria. Most cafés, shopping centres and so on will allow you to make up a fresh bottle if you take milk and a sterilized bottle with you.

FEEDING YOUR BABY

All babies, whether breast- or bottle-fed, need to feel warm and comforted while they are feeding. Your baby will soon look forward to his bottle-feeds as times when you cuddle him close. Feeds are not just for satisfying hunger. Your baby uses his mouth to explore the world, and sucking will provide him with a good deal of pleasure and comfort. So don't rush feeds; think of them as a time you can enjoy together.

Find a comfortable spot to sit and relax. Babies are super-sensitive to anxiety and tension. Some babies fuss and cry at first. So hold and rock your baby, and talk to him gently to help relax him. Support your baby's head in the crook of your arm and hold the bottle so that the teat is full of milk, to prevent him swallowing bubbles of air.

Your baby will probably want to pause once or twice to bring up wind. Either support him with his head resting between your thumb and forefinger, or put him on your shoulder and gently pat or rub his back until he burps. If he doesn't bring up some wind within a few minutes don't worry. Some babies hardly ever need to burp, and others bring it up later.

Never leave your baby alone with the bottle, as he could choke. If you are unavoidably interrupted during a feed, put the baby down, cover the bottle with its cup, and feed him when you are free again.

Four tips for happy bottle-feeding

- *Sterilize all feed equipment thoroughly.* You can choose between boiling, using a sterilizing fluid or tablets, or the new steam method. You will probably find it more convenient to prepare the sterilizing solution early in the morning or before you go to bed, and simply slip the used feeding equipment into it as you use it. Always make up a fresh solution each day.
- Make yourself comfortable before feeding. Collect together everything you will need, plus a drink or snack for yourself to help you relax, tissues to mop up spills, a clean nappy, and so on. Sit in a comfortable chair. You may find you need to lie your baby on a pillow to bring him up to the correct height, or rest your feet on a footstool or pile of books. Support your back with a cushion if necessary.
- *Try to give most of the feeds yourself in the early days.* At first you and your baby are getting to know each other, and feeding is an ideal time to do so. Don't hand your baby round like a parcel to be fed by other people. Of course you may like to share feeding with your baby's father if possible, and if you are going out or returning to work, whoever is looking after your baby can give him feeds.
- *Let your baby take as much as he wants.* Today's formulas are designed for demand feeding. Let your baby take as much as he needs to satisfy him. If he finishes his whole bottle, you can offer a little more. If there is some left in the bottom of the bottle at the end of a feed don't force him to finish it. Always discard any milk left after a feed.

STERILIZING BOTTLES

All feeding equipment should be sterilized until your baby is at least six months old. Go for wide-necked bottles that are easy to clean, and change teats frequently.

Always wash bottles immediately after feeding so as to remove all traces of milk. Use hot soapy water, and scrub the bottles with a bottle brush. Turn the teats inside out and clean thoroughly, rubbing inside with a little table salt to remove all deposits of milk. Rinse thoroughly in fresh warm water.

If you are using a sterilizing solution immerse the clean bottle in it, making sure that all equipment is fully immersed and that there are no air bubbles, which could lead to unsterilized patches. Keep the bottles and other equipment in the solution until you need it. When you take out the bottles rinse them with boiled water not tap water. Experts recommend that you do not use domestic microwave ovens for sterilizing.

If you are using the boiling method, boil bottles and caps for ten minutes and teats for three. Then put the caps on the bottles until they are ready to be used.

If you are using one of the new steam sterilizers read the instructions carefully and follow them exactly.

By the time your baby is between six months and one year old, depending on how active he has become, you can stop sterilizing. By this time he will have built up some resistance to germs, and if he has started crawling he will no doubt be picking up all sorts of things from the floor in any case. However, you should still make sure that all feeding equipment is carefully washed then dried with a clean kitchen towel before being stored in a clean, dry cupboard away from pets or flies.

QUESTIONS AND ANSWERS ABOUT BOTTLE-FEEDING

Q. *How do I know if my baby is getting enough?*
A. Modern baby milks are easily digested and absorbed, so your baby will feed on demand, just like a breast-fed baby. Feed your baby if he wakes and seems hungry, rather than trying to make him wait until feed time. It will be convenient to make up the same amount of milk in each bottle, but don't worry if he doesn't finish it. Most babies will take in roughly the same amount of milk each day, but at some mealtimes he will be hungrier than others, just like you. A rough rule of thumb is 65 g (2½ oz) of baby milk for every 500 g (1 lb) of his weight. As he gains weight the amount he takes will increase accordingly. So long as your baby is bright and alert with a pink, firm, healthy-looking skin, and is gaining weight regularly, you can be sure he is getting enough.

Q. *My baby is three months old and very fretful. Should I put him on solids?*
A. Experts advise that baby milk is sufficient to meet a baby's needs for the first three to six months of life. Try increasing the amount of milk you give him before introducing solids. Remember he could be bored or lonely rather than hungry. After the first few weeks your baby will not want to sleep all the time. Include him in family activities and take him out in the pram for walks. A sleepy baby is not necessarily a satisfied one. You can have your baby weighed regularly at the clinic to reassure you that he is growing as he should. And you can also talk to your health visitor to clear up any worries you have about his growth and

health. If hunger does seem to be the cause, cautiously introduce a few solid foods (see Chapter two) bearing in mind that these early 'tastes' are only intended to get him used to the feel and texture of solid food.

Q. *My baby seems to be very windy. Is there anything I can do?*
A. Excess wind may be caused by your feeding technique or by leaving him to cry and swallow air before feeding. Make sure that the teat is full of milk and that your baby doesn't get any air bubbles. Hold your baby slightly propped up, and release the teat occasionally so he can come up for air. Breast-fed babies naturally pause during their sucking several times during a feed. It might help to make the holes in the teat larger.

Q. *My baby is constipated. What should I do?*
A. First of all be sure it is constipation. It doesn't matter how infrequently your baby has a bowel motion, so long as when it comes it is soft. Bottle-fed babies do tend to be more prone to constipation than breast-fed ones, however. If the stool is hard and your baby has to strain to pass it, this is constipation. Try giving him extra water to drink between feeds. Some babies are especially prone to constipation in hot weather, when they need extra fluids to replace those lost in sweating. Offering your baby prune juice or any other fruit juice may also do the trick.

Q. *My baby is sick after every feed. How can I help?*
A. Lots of babies bring up a small amount of milk after each feed, often when they burp. Such possetting, as it is called, is quite normal and harmless. As long as your baby is well and gaining weight there is no need to worry. Simply arm yourself with a cloth to wipe up any spills before beginning the feed. If your baby has a tendency to be very sicky, try feeding him little and often, and hold him in an upright position to allow his feed to settle a little after he has had his feed. If the problem persists, see your doctor or health visitor.

Q. *I want to change from breast to bottle. How do I do it?*
A. If you have been fully breast-feeding, change over to the bottle gradually over a couple of weeks to allow both your breasts and the baby time to adjust. Start by dropping one breast-feed every couple of days, and substituting a bottle of baby milk until you are down to just one breast-feed a day. Daytime feeds are the easiest to drop. You or your

baby may like to carry on with one breast-feed for comfort, but if your baby is happy with his bottle then you can drop this last breast-feed as soon as it is convenient.

THE LAST BOTTLE

Your baby will have become very attached to his bottle over the months. There is no great hurry to wean him off it, even after he is well-established on solids. Give him the chance to drink from a cup or a beaker from the age of about six months, but don't force him to abandon his much-loved bottle if he enjoys having it, say, before he goes to bed, or when he first wakes up. So long as you do not give him sweet drinks in it, it will not harm his teeth. Sucking remains an important comfort to your baby all through the first year, and sometimes into his second or even third. Your baby may well like to keep on with a last bottle when he is tired or upset, or to help him relax. If you chat to other parents you will probably discover that many babies continue with their bottles well into the second or third year. Bear with him, and don't worry. He will give it up in his own good time.

2 STARTING SOLIDS

The age at which your baby will be ready to go on to solids is highly
individual. Few babies need solids before three months, while many
thrive quite happily on milk alone for six months. Boys especially often
seem hungrier and grow faster, so may be ready for solids earlier. If your
baby is breast-fed, her weight gain will start to slow after the age of
about three months – this is a normal, healthy pattern.

Fashions in weaning come and go. At one time mothers were advised
to add a little cereal to babies' bottles as early as two weeks of age. It is
now known that starting solids this early is unnecessary and harmful. A
tiny baby's digestive system is not mature enough to cope with anything
other than milk. Too-early solids can overload a baby's kidneys, leading
to dangerous dehydration, and may also set up infections and allergies,
or lead to obesity in later life.

Experts recommend that babies should be started on solids between

---

Ready for solids?

Your baby may be ready for solids if:

- She is at least three months old.
- She weighs (6–7 kg) 14–15 lb.
- She is putting things in her mouth.
- She shows an interest in what you are eating.
- She can keep a runny purée in her mouth without pushing it all out
  again.

Remember:

- Be guided by your baby. Just because your neighbour's baby is having
  solids, doesn't mean it is right for your baby.
- Some babies take to solids as early as three months, others not until a few
  months later.
- Your baby's main food is still milk, so it does not matter if there are some
  things she does not like.
- If your baby shows little interest, cries or refuses absolutely to take solids,
  she may not be ready yet. Leave it a week or so then try again.
- If you start too soon your baby may gag and be put off solids.
- Too-early solids can dull your baby's appetite for milk and stress her
  system.

the ages of about three and six months, though there are no hard and fast rules and the time varies from baby to baby. In order to benefit from solids your baby must have reached a stage in her development where she is capable of taking food from a spoon and is showing an interest in foods other than milk. Her digestive system also needs to be mature enough to cope with foods other than milk. Try not to delay introducing solids much beyond six months. If you leave it too long she may find it difficult to learn to take food from a spoon. However, the amount of solid food your baby consumes at first is only small. So as long as your baby's weight gain is satisfactory, don't rush things if she doesn't show any interest in solids. Try again a little later.

HOW TO BEGIN

Your baby has been used to a liquid diet, so at first she will prefer bland, sloppy foods. Start with a special baby rice cereal, mixed with either a little expressed breast milk, baby milk or boiled water. If there is a history of food allergy in your family avoid products containing gluten, such as wheat-based cereals, to begin with, as these might trigger off allergies. Other suitable first foods are mashed banana, unsweetened fruit purée such as apple or pear, or cooked vegetable purées such as potato or carrot. As your baby gets more used to solids you can try a wider variety of foods. Introduce new foods gradually, leaving two or three days between adding new tastes, so it is easy to identify any foods that upset her. If your baby does not like a particular food, simply leave it off the menu for a week or so and then try again. The chances are that she will accept it.

Try to cultivate a calm, relaxed attitude towards weaning. If your baby senses that you are tense she will be more likely to resist this new experience. Your aim is to show her that food is fun and there are plenty of new experiences for her to explore.

You can serve food either cold or warm. Test a little of the food on your wrist to make sure it is not too hot – it should feel neither hot nor cold.

Introduce solids at a feed when your baby is usually happy and relaxed: the midday feed or early evening one is often suitable. If your baby is out of sorts for any reason, delay introducing solids until she is back to her usual self. Take the edge off her hunger by giving her one breast, or half her bottle-feed. Before sitting down, make up a few teaspoonfuls of solid food in a small, non-breakable bowl. It should have the consistency of a thick, but runny soup. There is no need to sterilize feeding utensils, but they should be washed separately in very hot water, and you should wash your hands before preparing the food.

Once your baby has had half her milk feed, sit her on your lap or in her baby chair. Using a small, shallow spoon – a special plastic weaning spoon or a salt spoon is ideal – offer her a small amount of the food. She will probably be puzzled about what to do with it at first, so give her time. Don't push the spoon too far back into her mouth or she may gag, which could discourage her. As she tries to work out how to take the food, she may push it out with her tongue. This is quite usual. Simply scrape the food off her lips and let her try again. At first she will suck

---

What food?

At four to five months old:

- Stewed apple
- Puréed soft pear
- Stewed peaches
- Stewed apricots
- Cooked and puréed carrot, cauliflower, potato, peas, parsnip or leeks
- Baby rice mixed with breast milk, baby milk or boiled water
- Other gluten-free cereals

At six to seven months old:

- Hard-boiled egg yolk sieved and mixed with baby milk or breast milk
- Cooked chicken breast, puréed with breast milk, baby milk or boiled water, or a little liquid in which the meat was cooked
- Puréed lean beef (not bought mince)
- Smooth lentil or butter bean purée (skins removed first)
- Natural yoghurt with a little fruit purée

Don't give your baby:

- Food with salt, sugar or spices added
- Fatty meats: lamb and pork are too fatty at this stage
- Smoked or salted foods e.g. bacon, salami, yeast extract
- Shellfish, nuts or chunky peanut butter
- Fruit (dried or fresh) that has seeds
- Coffee, tea or alcohol
- Egg before she is six months old
- Anything with gluten before she is six months old. Gluten is wheat protein found in bread, rusks, wheat-based cereals, and anything made with flour

the food off the spoon. Once she has had enough she will turn her head away, or she may cry. Don't force your baby to take food if she seems reluctant. Let her have the rest of her breast- or bottle-feed, and try again a day or so later. Remember that her main nourishment at this stage still comes from milk, so there is no hurry.

Don't worry about the quantity of food either. These early tastes are just that; she has to find out that they are food.

THE NEXT STEP

Once your baby has learnt how to take food from a spoon and is beginning to enjoy it, you can introduce a wider variety of textures and tastes. At first you can mix new foods with baby rice. Gradually start to offer solids at other times of the day, so that eventually your baby is having three 'meals' corresponding to breakfast, lunch and tea. As you do this you can gradually build up the amount of food she has. Of course she will still be having a breast- or bottle-feed in the morning and before she goes to bed. There are some suggested weaning schedules on pages 32–5, but remember that these are not hard and fast rules. Be guided by your baby.

As your baby begins to get more of her nourishment from solids you can consider dropping one of her milk feeds, although milk still provides a good many nutrients after the age of six months. Don't be surprised if your baby's appetite changes in fits and starts. Some weeks she may want fewer solids and more milk. If she is ill she may become more babyish and want all her food from breast or bottle again. If you are breast-feeding you can soon rebuild your supply by frequent feeding.

NEW TASTES AND TEXTURES

By the time your baby is six or seven months old you can start adding a wider range of tastes and textures to her daily menus. By six months, whether or not your baby has teeth, she is able to chew. She delights in putting everything into her mouth. Exploit this tendency by giving her a wide variety of different textures, not just bland purées. After this age babies often become fussy, and refuse to eat food with lumps in it. Mash or finely mince her food, and let her have a spoon to hold while you are feeding her, so that she can experiment with feeding herself. Of course, she will make a mess, so protect the floor with newspapers or a large sheet of plastic. At six to seven months your baby may like to try some meat or fish. Poach a chicken breast or fish fillet in a little milk or water then mash or mince it, making certain there are no bones. Your baby may also like to try some cheese – choose a mild-flavoured one, or cottage cheese, and avoid smoked, blue or processed cheese. It is sensible to continue giving one new food at a time so that you can pinpoint any unusual reaction.

When you first start giving your baby lumpier food she may seem surprised by the change of texture, or even gag. Stay calm and encourage her to try the new food. She will soon learn to cope with it. As she progresses with solids, you can start giving her a savoury first course followed by a fruit purée or yoghurt for pudding. To prevent your baby developing a sweet tooth, avoid sweetened desserts except as an occasional special treat.

By eight months your baby may be having a two-course lunch followed by a drink of diluted fruit juice or plain water. She could also have a small meal at teatime, for instance a sandwich, plus some fruit, fruit yoghurt, or baby cereal and fruit purée, followed by a drink of milk from a cup.

FINGER FOODS

Even a baby who dislikes lumpy foods will love finger foods. Exploit her natural curiosity and her desire to put everything into her mouth by

Suggested finger foods

- Small cubes of cooked vegetables
- Rusks
- Toast fingers
- Celery (with any stringy bits removed)
- Pieces of red and green pepper
- Slices of peeled apple or pear
- Pieces of skinned, deseeded tomato
- Florets of cooked cauliflower
- Cubes of cheese
- Dates, dried apricots, sultanas, dried apples
- Miniature sandwiches – try fillings of soft cheese, smooth (not crunchy) peanut butter, chopped egg, savoury spreads, sugarless fruit spreads
- Tiny meatballs
- Slices of hardboiled egg
- Cubes of cooked, firm fish
- Cooked pasta shells or shapes, macaroni cheese
- Puffed wheat, rice crispies
- A smooth chicken bone with a few scraps of meat still clinging to it

offering her foods with which she can easily feed herself. Cooked peas, small cubes of cooked carrot, cubes of mild cheese, miniature sandwiches, slices of banana, fish fingers, or soft pasta shells are all ideal. At first she may play with more than she eats, but gradually she will learn to feed herself. Try not to mind if your baby plays with her food. Patting, tasting, turning her bowl upside down, are all part of her natural desire to explore the world and see how things work. You will deal with this messy but temporary stage better if you make sure her high chair is well away from your pretty wallpaper. Provide your baby with a stout bib, protect nearby furniture and carpets, and let her play. She is less likely to develop feeding problems later if you don't interfere too much. After all, it is not so awful if she dirties her clothes – or herself. As she gets older your baby will become more civilized.

DRINKS

Once your baby has got used to taking solids, you can start to introduce drinks into her new regime. Breast milk or baby milk will still provide most of her nourishment, but it is a good idea to get her used to drinking from a cup. Boiled water is thirst quenching (there is no need to boil it after your baby is six months old) or, if she doesn't like plain water, try adding a little fruit juice. Avoid baby syrups, as they tend to be sugary. 15 ml (½ fl oz) fruit juice to 30–60 ml (1–2 fl oz) water is about the right dilution. From about six months old your baby can start having drinks from a cup. It is probably easier for her, and kinder on your floor, if you use a spouted cup to start off with. However, if you let her practice with a small egg cup or the teat cover from her bottle she will master drinking from a cup sooner, so that if you go to visit someone and forget her beaker she is able to manage. Some babies do not appear to drink very much. So long as her nappies are wet whenever you change her and she doesn't appear to be constipated she is probably absorbing enough fluid for her needs from her food.

As your baby's solid feeding progresses you can change from breast or baby milk to ordinary cow's milk. Don't do this before six months, as your baby's immature kidneys cannot cope. In fact it may be better to wait if you can until she is a year old. If there is asthma or eczema in your family, it is certainly better to wait until then.

So long as the milk is pasteurized, there is no need to boil it. Don't give a child under five skimmed milk, as it does not contain all the essential nutrients. You will find that as your baby eats more solid food her demand for milk will decrease. However, milk is a food too, and if she has a milk drink before or with her meal she may take fewer solids. If this is the case, try substituting a drink of water or diluted fruit juice. It is probably best to give her her drink after the meal; and if you give her water it has the advantage of helping wash any food residues off her teeth and gums.

ADVANCED WEANING

As your baby gets used to solids she will probably enjoy joining in some of the family meal times, and this should be encouraged. But don't force her to sit with you until everyone has finished. If she has finished her own meal and wants to leave the table, let her do so.

Once you know which foods your baby likes and dislikes and if any upset her, you can start combining several foods. Casseroles are nourishing, and if you are preparing one for the rest of the family you can take a little out before you add any seasoning, purée it and give some to the baby. Don't add stock cubes. The food may taste bland to you but that is how your baby likes it.

Between about nine months and one year old your baby will probably have progressed to three solid meals a day. Include something from each of the different food groups each day (see pages 62–4) to ensure that she is getting a good balance of foods. If she doesn't like something, or it upsets her, simply substitute something from the same food group. There is no need to fret if she doesn't eat a particular food. No one food is vital or forbidden.

Your baby will probably still like to suck from the breast or bottle once or twice a day, and so long as you don't mind, there is no reason why she should not continue to do so for as long as you both feel happy with this.

HOMEMADE OR READY-PREPARED FOOD?

Commercial baby foods are ideal for those first few tastes of solids. They can be made up in small quantities and save hours of preparation. However, it is a good idea to get your baby used to the taste of fresh, home-prepared food too, so that she can join in with family meals and does not become hooked on the taste and texture of bought baby foods.

Making your own baby food is certainly cheaper, and has the added advantage that you know what is in it. Bought baby foods, on the other hand, have been processed to make them suitable for storing, and many contain additives such as cereal, sugar, flavouring agents and extra nutrients, which have been added to replace those lost during manufacture.

However, it is probably a counsel of perfection to suggest that you use only home-prepared food. Manufactured baby foods are handy, especially when you are away from home. They are quick to prepare, and fortunately they are now made to the highest standards.

You can have the best of both worlds by giving your baby a mixture of homemade and bought baby food. Do encourage your baby to eat a wide variety of foods. Read the labels so that you can pick the ones with the most nutritional value. By the time your baby is about 15 months old you should not need to use the commercial variety except in the occasional emergency.

WHAT TO LOOK OUT FOR IN COMMERCIAL BABY FOODS

- Check the amount of sugar in the product. Remember that glucose, sucrose, fructose and lactose are all forms of sugar. Ideally go for those that are sugar-free.
- Read the labels: ingredients are listed in order of the largest quantity first, so do not buy anything that has sugar (or water) first.
- Salt is rarely used in baby foods these days, but avoid products that list monosodium glutamate (MSG).
- Manufacturers operate a voluntary ban on colourings in baby foods, and most baby foods are also free of artificial additives. Those that are used are thought to be safe, but if you want to avoid them entirely you will need to read the label carefully (see pages 84–8). Don't just rely on the product being labelled additive-free.
- Many baby foods contain modified or purified starch – this helps bulk them out, and provides energy, but only in the form of empty calories with no nutritional value.
- If you have a family history of allergies choose products that are gluten free, and egg and milk free. Sometimes this will be clear from the label. Otherwise you will need to look at the list of ingredients.
- Avoid buying 'mixed dinners', as they usually contain a lot of empty

starch. If you want to combine meat and vegetables it is best to buy them separately and mix them yourself.

- Don't store unused food in tins. Transfer leftovers to a covered bowl and store in the fridge, for no longer than 48 hours.
- Don't feed your baby straight from the jar unless she is going to eat the entire contents. Germs from her saliva could contaminate the food. If you think she is not going to finish the whole jar, put the appropriate amount in her bowl and store the remainder covered in the fridge.
- Throw unused leftovers away after two days.

FOOD PREPARATION TIPS

Nothing could be simpler than preparing food for your baby. There is a special pleasure to be gained from providing meals for her, and you can ensure that you use only the best and freshest ingredients.

Safety first

- Be careful not to give your baby anything she could choke on. Check that all bones are smooth and splinter-free. Don't give whole nuts, especially peanuts, which contain a poisonous toxin which is released into your baby's lungs if she chokes.
- Don't leave your baby alone when she is eating or drinking.
- If your baby does choke she will usually cough up the offending food. Give her a drink of water and comfort her. If she does not cough it up herself, hold her upside down and knock her firmly between the shoulder blades.
- Store food covered in the fridge.
- Make sure pets are kept well away from your baby's food at meal times.
- Always wash your hands before preparing food or feeding your baby. Avoid handling food if you have any sort of diarrhoea infection.
- Always make sure your baby is strapped into her high chair.

Fruit syrups

Many fruit syrups claim to be 'free of added sugar', but do read the labels before buying. Such products often contain fruit sugars or other sugars found naturally in food that are equivalent to as many as four teaspoons of table sugar. Such sugars can damage the tooth enamel, especially if the drink is given at bedtime, because less saliva is produced during sleep. Avoid using these drinks too often. Give them only with meals, and make sure your baby rinses her mouth with plain water, or clean her teeth afterwards.

- *Cooking specially for your baby.* Prepare a large casserole (remember no salt, stock cubes or added seasoning). Divide it into baby-sized portions and store in the freezer.
- *Family meals.* Cook an extra portion of your own meal, then mash or blend it and store until the next day.
- *Combining commercially made and homemade foods.* For instance add a little cooked meat, fish, grated cheese and so on to a packet of dried vegetable mix. Serve fresh puréed fruit with rice cereal.
- *Storage.* You can keep prepared meals in the fridge for up to 24 hours. After cooking, put the food into a clean container and cool rapidly. Reheat thoroughly. Small amounts can be heated in a cup placed in a pan of simmering water. Do not reheat more than once.
- *Microwave.* You can safely reheat food in the microwave, but be particularly careful to mix the food thoroughly afterwards (to avoid hot spots), and test the temperature before giving it to your baby. Follow the microwave instructions to the letter.
- *Freezing.* Put blended or mashed portions of cooked food into ice-cube trays, small pots with lids, or empty plastic tubs, wrapped in clingfilm to eliminate air. Alternatively, put small dollops of food on foil, wrap well and freeze. Do not keep frozen food for long periods. Once food has been defrosted, do not refreeze.
- *Hygiene.* Feeding bowls, spoons and so on should be washed well in very hot, soapy water. Run the water as hot as you can bear it, protecting your hands with rubber gloves if necessary. Scrub sieves, blender parts and so on with a long-handled brush.
- *Keep* cooked and uncooked food separate. Always wash fruit and vegetables, and don't leave food lying around the kitchen uncovered.
- *Don't* soak vegetables in water before cooking – vitamins will be lost in the water. Cook vegetables in a small amount of water in a saucepan with a tight-fitting lid. Use the excess cooking liquid to make stocks and gravies or to add moisture when blending or mashing, to ensure that nutrients lost in the water are used.
- *Serve* some fresh fruit and raw vegetables each day, but make sure you peel them, and remove any hard or stringy bits.
- *Do* bear in mind your baby's age and stage of development when preparing her food. A four-month-old should have food the consistency of a thick soup. A six-month-old can cope with a mash, with a few lumps. A nine-month-old will be able to manage quite lumpy food.

SUGGESTED WEANING SCHEDULE

AGE	FIRST FEED	BREAKFAST
3–4 months	Breast or bottle	Breast or bottle
5 months	Breast or bottle	2 teaspoons baby rice or baby cereal Breast or bottle
6 months	Breast or bottle	Small bowl baby rice, cereal or rusk in milk
6–7 months	Breast or bottle	Baby cereal or hard-boiled or poached egg with bread Breast or bottle

puree

6oz

6oz

Mashed

apron 30 oz per day. 12 × 2   12 × 3
*   = 24 oz   36*

LUNCH	TEA/SUPPER	LAST FEED

Breast or bottle *6 oz*
1–2 teaspoons fruit
   or vegetable purée
   or baby rice
	Breast or bottle
	
	6 oz
		Breast or bottle
		
		6 oz

2 teaspoons puréed
   vegetable, or soup,
   or commercial
   baby food
Breast or bottle
	Breast or bottle	Breast or bottle

Puréed casserole with
   vegetables,
Puréed fruit, or
   commercial
   dinner, puréed
   vegetables
Puréed fruit or
   commercial dessert
	Hard-boiled egg yolk
	   sieved and mixed
	   with formula or
	   breast milk, and
	   rusk, or mashed
	   banana
	Breast or bottle
		Breast or bottle

Mashed chicken, fish
   or calves' liver or
   pulses, with
   mashed potato,
   mashed peas and
   gravy, or
   commercial dinner
   plus vegetable
Mashed ripe pear,
   banana or fruit
   dessert
Water or diluted fruit
   juice
	Mashed cauliflower
	   cheese, or cheese
	   sandwich, or pasta
	   with cheese, or
	   yoghurt and fruit
	Breast or bottle, or
	   diluted fruit juice,
	   or milk from a cup
		Breast or bottle
		low fat
		or cottage cheese

SUGGESTED WEANING SCHEDULE – *Contd.*

AGE	FIRST FEED	BREAKFAST
7–8 months	Breast or bottle	Baby cereal or Weetabix and milk, fruit, wholemeal toast and butter or margarine Milk from cup
9–12 months	Breast or bottle if wanted	Baby cereal or Weetabix and milk, or hard-boiled or poached egg, toast Diluted fruit juice

N.B. This is only a suggested schedule. Be prepared for setbacks, and be guided by your baby's individual needs. It is impossible to be rigid about ages or specific amounts, since every baby is different. As you gradually increase the amount of solids, your baby's appetite for milk will lessen, and she will satisfy her thirst from water and fruit juice

QUESTIONS AND ANSWERS ABOUT WEANING

Q. *I've tried giving my four-month-old some baby rice but every time I do so she gags and turns her head away. What should I do?*
A. It is quite usual for a baby to grimace or shudder at her first tastes of

LUNCH	TEA/SUPPER	LAST FEED
Chicken casserole, mashed potato and tomatoes, or mashed spaghetti bolognese, or bean casserole, or commercial meal Milk jelly or stewed fruit, or commercial dessert Water or diluted fruit juice	Wholemeal cheese sandwiches, or cheese on toast Milk from a cup	Breast or bottle
Chopped meat or fish with vegetables, or pasta or risotto, or commercial dinner Piece of fruit or yoghurt, or ready made dessert Water or diluted fruit juice	Baked beans on toast, or fish fingers and bread and butter or margarine, or slice of quiche, or homemade pizza Piece of fruit Water or diluted fruit juice, or milk from a cup	Breast or bottle, if wanted, or milk from a cup

instead of just milk. However, milk is still an excellent balanced source of nutrients. You can continue to give the breast or bottle for the whole of the first year, or even longer if it suits you both.

solid food. And as she attempts to bite, chew and swallow, some coughing or gagging is also normal. Your baby may be gagging because you have made up her food too thick – it should be runny, about the consistency of thick soup. Alternatively you may be offering her more than she can cope with. Place about a quarter of a teaspoon on the tip of a shallow spoon to start off with, and place the spoon just inside her mouth; you may be pushing it too far back. Don't ever try to force your baby to take food she doesn't want. If she has to take more than she needs she'll only spit it up. It may be best to leave solids for a couple of weeks and then try again, bearing these points in mind.

Q. *My six-month-old baby doesn't seem to like solids. Any hints?*
A. Most babies are probably ready for solids between four and six months. Try leaving off solids for a week or so, and then try again. When you do so take it slowly. Milk is still a vital part of your baby's diet for the whole of the first year, and so long as she is still having her breast or bottle she is getting plenty of nourishment. You may feel

INTRODUCING SOLIDS – AT-A-GLANCE GUIDE

Food	4 to 6 months
Cereal e.g. baby rice	Start gluten free
Fruit	
Vegetables	
Finger foods	
Well-cooked mashed or chopped food from the family menu without added salt or sugar	
Juice from a beaker	

happier giving her a vitamin supplement to ensure that she doesn't run short of any essential nutrients. Consult your health visitor for advice.

Q. *My eight-month-old baby won't eat anything lumpy.*
A. By about six months old your baby should be able to chew. She will prefer brightly coloured, interesting-looking food to a brown mush, so make separate little piles of cooked, bright carrot, peas, and meat or cheese, and let her feed herself. Her natural curiosity and desire to try out new things should take care of the rest. Given the opportunity, she will learn to chew and cope with textured food. But if your baby senses that you are anxious or worried she may feel nervous herself. Finger foods usually go down well with this age group. Let her join in family

6 to 8 months	9 to 12 months
Carefully introduce cereals containing gluten	Family cereals
Mashed, sieved or puréed	Gradually replace with food from family menu
Mashed, sieved or puréed	Gradually replace with chopped, well-cooked vegetables
Give large finger foods that baby can grasp in palm of hand	Introduce small finger food, e.g. peas, squares of cheese
	Start offering food from family menu
	Start

mealtimes too; her natural desire to be a part of the family will encourage her to eat up.

Q. *My ten-month-old won't drink from a cup.*
A. So long as your baby is producing wet nappies, she is probably getting enough liquid from her food and from her breast or bottle. Provide a spouted cup of juice or water at meal times, but don't force her to drink. Check her beaker to make sure the liquid isn't flowing from it too fast, as this may be alarming for her. You could also try a small cup or egg cup, so that she can sip small quantities. It could be that your baby just loves sucking. Most babies still have a strong need to suck at this age, and there is no need to wean her from breast or bottle until she is a year old or even older. Rather than let it become an issue, you could forget all about her cup for a while then reintroduce it, or a different one, in a few weeks' time.

Q. *My seven-month-old baby went back to complete breast-feeding during a recent illness. Is this OK?*
A. It is quite normal for a baby to want to go back to breast- or bottle-feeding when she is ill. Sucking is a great source of comfort for your baby. Once she is feeling better she will regain her interest in solid food.

Q. *Since my baby has been on solids her nappies smell nasty. Is this normal?*
A. Unfortunately, yes. A breast-fed baby's bowel motions are usually inoffensive, but once she starts on solids or fresh milk her stools do start to smell. So long as they are not watery or exceptionally foul smelling, there is no reason to worry. If they become diarrhoea, of course, you should take her to the doctor.

Q. *Why does my baby have such a small appetite?*
A. It is possible that your baby needs less than you think she does. Your baby's weight gain slows down in the second half of the first year. Given a reasonable selection of food, no child will starve herself. So long as your baby is bright and lively, and has plenty of wet nappies, she is probably getting enough food. It could be that your baby is still getting a great deal of nourishment from milk, and this is quenching her appetite for other foods. Babies also go through growth spurts. Perhaps temporarily she needs less, but this period of eating little will

HOW YOUR BABY'S DEVELOPMENT AFFECTS HER EATING HABITS

Age	Reflex	Abilities
1 to 3 months	Rooting, sucking and swallowing reflexes	Sucks milk from breast or bottle
4 to 6 months	Rooting reflex fades	Becomes more efficient at sucking Begins to be able to chew Grasps objects with whole hand Grips objects, puts them to her mouth and bites
7 to 9 months	Gag reflex becomes less developed with chewing of solids	More sophisticated chewing movements develop Sits up on own Develops ability to let go of objects Can hold bottle herself Begins to be able to grasp with fingers
10 to 12 months		Reaches for spoon Bites crunchy foods Grasps bottle and foods and brings them to her mouth Can drink from a cup that is held Able to lick food from lower lip Finer finger movement enables her to pick up smaller morsels

probably be followed by a time when she wants to eat everything in sight. So long as your baby enjoys her food it doesn't matter how much or how little she eats.

Q. *My baby is five months old and all she will eat is chocolate pudding. What can I do?*
A. In the early days of weaning it is common for babies to prefer sweet things. Babies seem to have a natural preference for sweet foods, probably because breast milk is fairly sweet. Try not to get too anxious about your baby's eating habits, as this will transmit itself to her and make feeding a miserable business for both of you. Persevere with a variety of unsweetened and savoury foods, but don't make a fuss if she refuses to be tempted. Simply take the food away and try again another time. You will find that in a month or so she will enjoy a good mix of tastes. Incidentally there is no reason why she shouldn't have the occasional chocolate pudding as a treat.

Q. *My baby, who is ten months old, has always been fussy, so we started coaxing her to eat. Now every meal time has become a battleground, and she won't eat a thing unless we turn it into a game. I'm sure she can't be getting a balanced diet.*
A. One of the commonest problems parents encounter is a baby's refusal to eat what they think is a balanced diet. In fact there is no one food your baby has to have, and so long as you present her with a good variety of food she is probably getting what she needs. Studies have shown that, offered a range of foods, babies automatically take in the correct quantities of the various nutrients, though this is likely to be over several days, or even weeks. There is no harm in making feeding time into a game occasionally, but it can be a terrible bind if you have to spend every meal time bribing her to eat. The best way to avoid this is to be quite calm and matter-of-fact. Present her with a range of finger foods, so that she has control over what she eats. But if she doesn't eat simply take the food away without fuss and wait until next meal time. Let your baby eat with the family, if she is not already doing so, and try to make those meal times happy, sociable occasions. With this approach your baby won't necessarily eat everything she is offered, but it will take some of the tension out of meal times.

3 YOUR TODDLER – FIT FOR THE FUTURE

By the time your baby has reached the age of one year he is a real part of the family. In order to grow strong and healthy his body needs over 50 different nutrients. The best way to meet these needs is to provide him with a varied diet which contains enough protein, carbohydrates, fats, vitamins, minerals and trace elements. But there are important differences between a healthy diet for an adult and a healthy diet for a child. Children need more protein and energy in relation to their size than adults, and they also need more of certain vitamins and minerals in order to meet their growth and energy needs.

All this may sound rather daunting, so it is reassuring to know that you can meet these needs quite simply by ensuring that your child eats a wide range of different foods. It helps to think in terms of food groups rather than specific foods. And especially if your child develops food fads – a common phenomenon between the ages of one and three – it is important to bear in mind that there is no one food that is vital. If your child doesn't like a particular food, simply substitute another food from the same group to meet his needs.

The keynote is variety, and that means ensuring that he gets a mix of raw and cooked foods; high calorie and low calorie; chewy, crisp and soft; sharp and mild; fresh and processed. It means varying your cooking techniques too: don't just fry everything, or your child will get too much fat; instead boil, steam, casserole, grill, stir fry or serve raw. This way food becomes fun for both your child and you.

How much your child eats will vary depending on how much he moves about. Your toddler's growth slows down after his first birthday, but he will still have growth spurts from time to time – a common one is around about the time he starts to walk. It is perfectly normal for a child to eat everything in sight one day and pick at his meals like a sparrow the next. So long as your child's height and weight are within the limits for his age (see page 72), there is no need to worry about this. A calm, matter-of-fact acceptance of these variations in appetite is the way to cope. The same goes for food binges, when your child seems to live exclusively on just a few foods. Again, this is quite normal at this age. So long as your child is happy, healthy and growing, it is likely that he is eating all he needs.

WHAT FOOD SHOULD YOUR CHILD EAT?

As stated above, variety is the key to ensuring your child receives what he needs. In the following pages you will find a rundown of the various nutrients and why they are important, but don't become too bogged down by the technical aspects. Milk remains an important part of your child's diet until he is five. It is high in protein and also calcium, the main constituent of growing bones. The fat in milk also carries vitamins, which is why you should give your child whole milk rather than skimmed until he is two. After that you may give him semi-skimmed milk if it fits in with your family eating habits better and as long as the rest of his diet is good. Follow these guidelines:

- Encourage your child to drink milk every day. Up to 600 ml (1 pint) is fine, but some children who drink more than this can lose their appetite for other foods, so discourage him from drinking too much. Incidentally if your child genuinely doesn't like milk, don't force it on him.
  You can offer him disguised milk in custard, yoghurts, pancakes and so on. He may eat other milk-based foods such as cheese with gusto. If you really cannot get him to take milk of any description (extremely unlikely) simply substitute other foods which will meet his needs for calcium and protein.
- Don't give cow's milk to a baby younger than one year old. Use a follow-on milk to bridge the gap from about six months of age.
- Always use pasteurized milk. Skimmed milk is not suitable, as the fat intake is reduced and your child might not get enough calories to meet his energy needs, since milk still forms a staple of his diet. Also, the fat in milk contains all-important vitamins.

It is best to think of milk as a food rather than a drink, and to continue to offer water or diluted fruit juice to quench thirst.

Your child needs protein at every meal and at least two servings each of fruit and vegetables each day. Exactly how much he will eat varies, but large portions can look daunting to a small child. As a general rule of thumb, offer him about a third of the amount you are having. He can always have more if he seems hungry.

PLANNING A MENU

Use the daily food plan below to help you plan nourishing meals and snacks for your child. Steer clear of empty calories in the form of sugary snacks, biscuits or sweets, and avoid fatty or salty foods. That is not to say that such foods should be banned altogether, but try to keep them as occasional treats to be eaten after something more nutritious. If your child is a faddy eater it is especially important not to let him fill up on sweets and snacks that could spoil his appetite for more nourishing food. One way to cope is to make snack foods part of the menu from

---

To help you plan a day's menu follow the following guidelines.

Provide one portion of each:

Breakfast
1. One high-protein food, e.g. egg, cheese, cereal and milk
2. Bread with butter or margarine
3. Milk
4. Fruit

Lunch
1. One high-protein food e.g. stew, grilled meat, fish, cheese, eggs or pulses, or casserole with potatoes
2. Vegetables – one cooked, one raw
3. Bread
4. Milk or yoghurt
5. Dessert – either based on mixture of milk, eggs, fruit or piece of fruit

Dinner
1. One high-protein food
2. Vegetables – one or two cooked, or one raw
3. Bread and butter, or potato
4. Milk
5. Dessert (see lunch)

Snacks
These should be nourishing and low in sugar and fat so as not to spoil your child's appetite, e.g. fruit juice with a cracker, rusk or slice of bread; small pieces of fruit; small pieces of raw vegetable, e.g. carrot sticks; cubes of cheese with slice of bread, or crispbread.

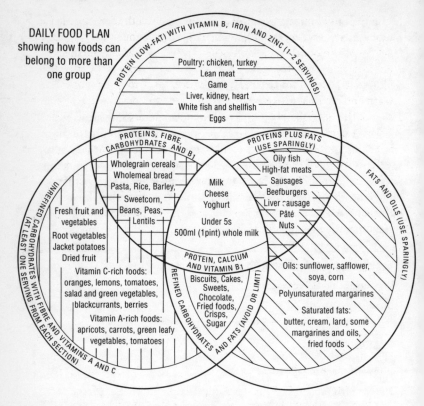

DAILY FOOD PLAN showing how foods can belong to more than one group

PROTEIN (LOW-FAT) WITH VITAMIN B, IRON AND ZINC (1-2 SERVINGS)

Poultry: chicken, turkey
Lean meat
Game
Liver, kidney, heart
White fish and shellfish
Eggs

PROTEINS, FIBRE, CARBOHYDRATES AND B1

Wholegrain cereals
Wholemeal bread
Pasta, Rice, Barley,
Sweetcorn,
Beans, Peas,
Lentils

PROTEINS PLUS FATS (USE SPARINGLY)

Oily fish
High-fat meats
Sausages
Beefburgers
Liver sausage
Pâté
Nuts

UNREFINED CARBOHYDRATES WITH FIBRE AND VITAMINS A AND C (AT LEAST ONE SERVING FROM EACH SECTION)

Fresh fruit and vegetables
Root vegetables
Jacket potatoes
Dried fruit

Vitamin C-rich foods:
oranges, lemons, tomatoes,
salad and green vegetables,
blackcurrants, berries

Vitamin A-rich foods:
apricots, carrots, green leafy
vegetables, tomatoes

Milk
Cheese
Yoghurt

Under 5s
500ml (1pint) whole milk

FATS AND OILS (USE SPARINGLY)

PROTEIN, CALCIUM AND VITAMIN B1

REFINED CARBOHYDRATES AND FATS (AVOID OR LIMIT)

Biscuits, Cakes,
Sweets,
Chocolate,
Fried foods,
Crisps,
Sugar

Oils: sunflower, safflower,
soya, corn

Polyunsaturated margarines

Saturated fats:
butter, cream, lard, some
margarines and oils,
fried foods

time to time. For example give him ice-cream for his pudding occasionally, or a little heap of crisps as part of his main meal.

Research has shown that toddlers prefer to eat little and often. Because of their tiny stomachs it is easier for them to cope with several smaller meals rather than the traditional adult pattern of three main meals a day. The way to deal with this without disrupting the entire family's eating pattern is to make nutritious snacks a part of your child's daily menu. It doesn't matter after all whether your child fills his protein needs from several snacks or from 'proper' meals – what counts is that he receives sufficient protein. You will find that your child automatically balances his intake over the course of several meals. In fact, parents of faddy eaters who complain that 'he never eats a thing' often find when they look at their child's total intake including snacks that it is quite adequate.

With this in mind plan snacks that form part of the total menu. Go
for fresh fruit and vegetables, sandwiches with peanut butter, cheese or
egg, rather than cakes, crisps, biscuits and other ready-made snacks.
Another reason to steer clear of such foods, of course, is the risk of
tooth decay. Each time you eat, small particles of food cling to your
teeth and are then broken down by saliva to form acids which attack
the tooth enamel. Sweet, stick foods and sugary drinks are the biggest
culprits when it comes to tooth decay. Watch for 'hidden' sugar in
baked beans, tomato ketchup, squash and so on. Encourage your child
to finish his meal or snack with a glass of plain water. Rather than
ending a meal with a sweet dessert, offer a piece of fruit, or better still a
piece of cheese, which helps counteract the effects of acids formed by
food breakdown on tooth enamel. And, of course, help your child
clean his teeth after eating.

MIXING AND MATCHING FOOD

Children prefer familiar foods. When introducing a new food, offer it
with something your child knows and likes. Don't worry if he doesn't
touch it or just plays with it the first time you offer something new. It is
all part of learning to accept it.

Many toddlers dislike dry foods and find them hard to eat. When
giving something dry, such as fish fingers or meat loaf, serve it with
something moist such as peas in white sauce, or baked beans.

The same goes for flavours. Sharp, acidic foods such as orange may go
down better when combined with a mild-flavoured food, for instance
slices of banana.

Bear in mind too that some foods are difficult for tiny, unskilled
hands to deal with. Peas or beans may be difficult to scoop up. Either let
your child pick them up with his fingers, or mix them with mashed
potatoes for easier eating. He may find spooning up soup tiring; why not
serve it in a mug so that he can drink it, or make it slightly thicker so it
does not spill out of the spoon so easily?

Your child will find it easier to eat with his fingers, so let him have
one or two finger foods with each meal. Mixed salads are more difficult
to cope with than separate heaps of raw vegetables. Take care over the
size of pieces of food. Serve your child bite-sized pieces for ease. Tiny,
bite-sized sandwiches usually go down well.

Think about the texture of your child's food. At each meal try

Sample menus for toddlers

One year old

Day 1

Breakfast Cereal, (e.g. porridge, baby muesli, puffed wheat, Weetabix) with milk
Slice of toast with margarine or butter
Fruit juice or piece of fruit

Mid-morning snack Cup of milk

Lunch Macaroni cheese with tomato and peas
Slices of apple or yoghurt
Water or fruit juice

Dinner Minced meat with carrots and potato
Rice pudding
Water or fruit juice

Bedtime Cup of milk

Day 2

Breakfast Boiled egg with wholemeal bread
Fruit juice or piece of fresh fruit (e.g. grapes, apple, fruits in season)
Milk

Mid-morning snack Cup of milk and plain biscuit

Lunch Baked beans on toast, peas, carrots or other green or yellow vegetable
Yoghurt and fruit
Diluted fruit juice or water

Mid-afternoon Cup of milk

Dinner Fish in sauce, broccoli and potato
Rusk
Fruit or fruit yoghurt

Bedtime Cup of milk

serving one soft food that slips down easily, one crisp food for easy chewing and crunchy enjoyment, and one chewy food to encourage chewing skills. Children often have difficulty with meat because of its stringy texture, which perhaps explains why hamburgers are so popular. Try mincing or casseroling meat rather than roasting or grilling.

STRIKING THE RIGHT BALANCE

When planning food for your toddler it is important to keep a balance. Doctors have recently identified a new syndrome: 'muesli belt malnutrition', brought about by parents applying the new diet rules too zealously. They have read that a high-fibre diet is a 'good thing'. However, it is possible to have too much of a good thing, and fibre is a

Sample menus for toddlers

18 months old

Day 1
Breakfast Boiled egg with wholemeal bread, spread with butter or margarine
Piece of fruit
Cup of milk

Mid-morning snack Fruit juice and plain biscuit

Lunch Liver pâté on wholemeal bread fingers
Slices of apple with raisins
Water or fruit juice

Dinner Grilled fish fingers with baked beans, mashed potato and tomato
Fruit and yoghurt

Bedtime Cup of milk

Day 2
Breakfast Cereal with milk, and wholemeal toast with margarine and sugar-free jam (not diabetic jam which may have artificial sugar and additives)
Piece of fruit
Cup of milk

Mid-morning snack Fruit juice and small banana

Lunch Wholemeal sandwich with smooth peanut butter
Slices of orange and kiwi fruit
Water, diluted fruit juice or milk

Dinner Casseroled chicken with carrots and potato
Stewed apple with custard

Bedtime Cup of milk

case in point. Fibre-rich food is both low-calorie and filling, which of course is why adults with weight problems can benefit from increasing their fibre intake. The trouble is that if a child eats too many high-fibre foods he feels full up before he has been able to take in the number of calories he needs – the result is malnutrition. It may seem incredible to talk about malnutrition in our affluent age, but the fact is that small children are actively growing and that means they need to eat highly nutritious foods that provide plenty of energy – what the experts call high-energy-density foods. If fat intake is cut and refined carbohydrates are avoided it can be hard to maintain the necessary energy intake in some young children.

Moreover, bran contains a substance that inhibits the body from absorbing trace minerals such as calcium, copper, iron, magnesium, phosphorous and zinc. Some experts have suggested that the body adapts to low mineral intakes but this has not yet been proved.

Sample menus for toddlers

Two to three years

Day 1

Breakfast   Porridge with milk
Wholemeal bread and savoury
spread (e.g. peanut butter, sesame
or sunflower)
Grapes
Milk

Lunch   Cheese and tomato pizza
Cress, grated carrot, grated beetroot
salad (or other salad vegetables as
liked)
Fruit and yoghurt
Diluted fruit juice or water

Dinner   Beef and vegetable
casserole
Apple snow
Milk

Day 2

Breakfast   Shredded wheat and
milk
Bread, butter or margarine and
sugar-free jam
Pear
Milk

Lunch   Egg and tomato sandwich
Fruit
Milk

Dinner   Roast lamb, baked potato,
broccoli
Banana mashed or sliced into
yoghurt
Fruit juice or water

Note: Don't add salt to your child's food at table, or sugar to his cereal or
drinks

Children need plenty of protein, which supplies approximately a
tenth of their energy needs. If your child's energy needs are not met
from other sources, protein is used for energy and is then not available
for growth needs. The answer is to apply a dash of commonsense. By all
means give your child plenty of fruit and vegetables, wholemeal bread
and cereals, but don't add extra bran to his food or give him foods that
contain added fibre.

The same applies to fats. It is better to give your toddler butter or a
polyunsaturated margarine than a low-fat spread. And buy full-fat
cheeses rather than the low-fat variety, to ensure he gets sufficient
calories.

Foods to avoid
Whole nuts, salted nuts
Crunchy peanut butter

Wholemeal bread with added bran, or very coarse bread with whole
grains
Very salty dishes
Very spicy foods, especially hot spices
Chinese food (often has added monosodium glutamate see pages 85–6)
Sweetened fizzy drinks, squashes etc.

HUNGER STRIKE! – HOW TO DEAL WITH A FADDY EATER

Food fads and food refusal are almost universal in the toddler years. The
best way to deal with this is to remain calm and matter-of-fact.
Remember that there is no one food that is vital for your child to have –
there is always an alternative. Use the daily food plan on page 44 and
at-a-glance food guide on page 82 to find nutritious foods that belong to
the same group.

You are likely to feel hard done by if you have spent hours cooking a
delicious meal only to have it rejected. Avoid feelings of resentment by
cooking foods you know your child enjoys. Be flexible about your
toddler's likes and dislikes and he will soon grow out of his faddiness. It
is when food is allowed to become an issue that meal-time battles
persist – often for years. Remember – and try to believe it – no healthy

---

Healthy eating tips for your toddler

- Give your child a good variety of different foods by choosing a wide
  selection from the different food groups.
- Buy fresh fruit and vegetables.
- Vary your cooking techniques.
- Present food attractively. Separate little piles of fresh, colourful foods
  look more appetizing than a brown mush.
- Don't worry too much if your child's diet seems to be unbalanced on any
  one day – it is what he eats over the course of several days or weeks that
  matters.
- Don't fuss or coax if your child refuses what you put in front of him.
- Buy high-quality protein foods – lean meat, fish, pulses and so on.
- Go easy on roughage. Don't add extra bran to food, and cook whole
  grains such as brown rice in plenty of water to make them more
  digestible.
- Don't add sugar or salt to food. Avoid hidden sugar in cakes, biscuits,
  drinks.

child has ever starved himself. If your child does not want to eat, simply remove the food, and wait until the next meal time. The chances are he will be ravenous.

If you are afraid that your child is not getting enough to eat, one useful way to put things into perspective is to keep a food diary. Note down everything he eats, including snacks, over the course of one or two weeks. You will probably be amazed at just how much he has eaten on average over the time you have kept the diary.

Tips on coping with a faddy eater

- Make as little fuss as possible if your child refuses food. It won't hurt him to miss the occasional meal.
- If you know that your child absolutely hates a particular food, don't serve him it. After all how would you feel if you were forced to eat something you really disliked? Remember there is always a substitute.
- Present food attractively: children especially like colour – for example a sprig of parsley, a dash of red tomato, a piece of carrot.
- Offer small portions. It is better to let him ask for second helpings than to overwhelm him with too large a plateful.
- Don't force your child to leave a clean plate.
- Don't worry about manners. If he wants to pick his food up in his fingers, let him. He'll grow out of it.
- Don't insist that he eats the savoury course before the dessert. So long as the dessert is a nourishing one, what does it matter which he eats first? He will develop more sociable eating habits as he gets older.
- Avoid empty-calorie snacks such as crisps, sweets and ice-cream between meals.
- Be careful over the timing of meals. A child who has to wait hours for his evening meal may be too tired to eat by the time it arrives. It may be better to provide him with a special tea earlier in the day. Conversely, if his meals are too close together he may not feel hungry.
- Don't coax, nag or threaten if he refuses to eat. Avoid bribing him, too. If he realizes his refusal to eat is bothering you, you are handing him a powerful weapon.
- Try not to rush him. It doesn't matter if he finishes after the rest of the family. Hurrying him will make him tense and loss of appetite will follow.

- Don't expect too much. It is unrealistic to expect a toddler to eat up everything with perfect table manners. Give him time.
- If your child has a small appetite, check how much he is drinking to make sure he isn't filling himself up so that he has no room for the rest of the meal. The toddler who has a drink of juice with him all day long is not going to eat very much.
- Be guided by your child. Children's appetites and needs vary enormously, just as adults' do. The slim, small child with a small appetite is just as likely to be healthy and fit as the child who wolfs down everything in sight.
- Try to avoid snacks between meals if he is not eating well at meal times.
- Give him the chance to try new foods but don't insist that he eats anything he doesn't like.
- Many toddlers dislike cooked vegetables. If this is the case offer him them raw.
- Involve your child in simple food preparation from time to time. Toddlers love to 'help'. Older toddlers can be allowed to 'choose' what they would like to eat – for example fish fingers or macaroni cheese for lunch.
- Try to keep his meals in a reasonable routine. It is also a good idea for him to get into the habit of always sitting up at the table or in his high chair whenever he has a snack or meal.
- Keep meal times fun.

SWEET SENSE

Sooner or later your child is going to discover sweets. If you have older children it will be harder to shield him from sweets than if he is your first child. Sweets can dull the appetite for more nourishing meals, cause obesity and, of course, tooth decay. Studies have shown that sweets eaten at meal times, when saliva is being plentifully produced, are far less harmful than when they are eaten between meals. Sweets are a source of empty calories, so if your child is going to have something sweet it is far better to give him something in which the natural sweetness is wrapped up in other nutrients and actually fills him up. For example, a banana or an apple will satisfy your child more than a sweet or a biscuit and will use up fewer calories, as well as providing him with fibre, vitamins and minerals. However, banning sweets altogether may not be the answer, as your child will come to feel deprived and may demand sweets even more. A few commonsense rules may help:

1. Encourage friends and relatives not to give sweets as presents. There are plenty of small, fun toys such as bubble mix, tiny notepads, dolls, soft toys, or books that are readily available and cost no more than a packet of sweets.
2. Don't use sweets as a reward, for example after he has had an injection, or as a treat for eating up his meal.
3. If your child must have sweets, encourage him to have them at a particular time, for instance on Saturday morning, or after dinner – and make sure he cleans his teeth afterwards. Incidentally some sweets are more likely to cause tooth decay than others. Sticky sweets that take a long time to chew and keep the teeth bathed in sugar are the worst villains in this respect, e.g. toffees or boiled sweets which stay in the mouth a long time. It is less harmful to give your child those that melt rapidly, e.g. jelly sweets or chocolate buttons.
4. Don't keep sweets in the house. Instead keep plenty of fresh fruit, dried fruit, and other wholesome, easily prepared foods.
5. Avoid emotionally loading sweets. If your child asks for sweets don't react with horror – buy him a packet casually. Encourage him to see other things, for example an exotic fruit, as treats too.
6. Ask your dentist about fluoride drops or tablets, and find out whether the water is fluoridated in your area. Fluoride helps strengthen the teeth and will help protect your child's permanent teeth.
7. Provide your child with an alternative such as an apple, banana or rusk *before* you reach the supermarket checkout with its tempting array of sweet goodies just within your toddler's reach.
8. Experiment with making your own sweets occasionally – your toddler can help. That way you know what goes in to the sweets and can make sure the sugar content is not too high.

QUESTIONS AND ANSWERS ABOUT FEEDING A TODDLER

Q. *My toddler won't eat his 'greens'. What can I do?*

A. First of all bear in mind that there is no one food your child has to

have. Many children dislike cooked cabbage. Why not try broccoli
instead? In a few weeks he will probably have forgotten that he didn't
like cabbage, and eat it enthusiastically. Many toddlers dislike the
texture of cooked vegetables. Try giving him them raw, such as sticks of
carrot or finely shredded cabbage, or stir frying them so that they retain
a little bite. And don't forget red and yellow vegetables like carrots,
sweetcorn and tomato. If he simply refuses all vegetables in whatever
shape or form, make sure he gets plenty of fruit and ask your health
visitor whether he should take vitamin drops.

Q. *My child eats perfectly when he goes to his granny's. But he constantly
plays with his food and refuses to eat it at home.*
A. Food faddiness often becomes more complicated when other
people, such as relatives, enter the picture. Try to keep calm, and not
to get worried, angry or guilty. Whatever you do, don't be tempted to
resort to bribery. Playing with food is common in the toddler years, and
it is best not to be too strict about it. Of course you can draw the line at
him throwing his meal on the floor or smearing it in his hair, but apart
from that, does it really matter if he makes a mess? Put a plastic sheet
on the floor. Allow him a reasonable time to finish his meal and then if
he still doesn't want it remove it without fuss.

Q. *My child will only eat processed food. Is there anything I can do?*
A. Toddlers are naturally contrary – it is part of their growing
independence. Often a toddler senses that you care more about food
you have spent hours preparing. One way round this is to combine
some processed foods with fresh ones. You can also make sure that you
make sensible choices when you buy processed foods, for instance
choose fruit tinned in natural fruit juice rather than syrup, and make
your own fruit yoghurt by chopping up cubes of apple or banana into
natural yoghurt. Hamburgers, fish fingers, baked beans and so on are
available additive free, so do read the labels. Go for thick-cut or
oven-baked chips rather than the crinkle-cut variety, which are
fattier.

Q. *How can I get my toddler to drink milk?*
A. The short answer is – you can't. But though milk is a convenient
way of ensuring that your child gets his protein and calcium rations,
there are other ways he can meet these needs. Try giving him milk in

custards, milk puddings and sauces, and adding it to mashed potato, pancakes or scrambled eggs. Cheese and yoghurt are just as nutritious as milk. Consult pages 57, 59 to find other sources of these nutrients.

Q. *My toddler will only eat mushy food. How can I encourage him to eat lumps?*
A. You can go along with his natural preferences by providing him with foods such as shepherd's pie, fish pie, scrambled eggs, smooth sauces, and milk puddings such as semolina. Provide finger foods with every meal to encourage him to experiment with different textures. Try not to fuss if he doesn't eat them.

4 FOOD FACTS

The problem for anyone with a family to feed is perhaps not so much a lack of information as too much – a lot of it confusing and contradictory. Most of us were brought up on a diet of meat and two vegetables, with lashings of cream and butter and eggs a daily treat. Today such a diet has been condemned by experts, who blame it for many illnesses such as heart disease, diabetes, digestive problems, bowel disorders and a whole host of other ailments that are rife in the West.

This chapter examines the nutritional content of various foods and explains their role in creating good health.

FATS

Weight for weight, fats are the highest-calorie food. They improve the flavour and texture of food, and help you to feel full and satisfied. Fat is most obviously contained in butter, lard, cheese and so on, but there is hidden fat in most foods – for example an egg contains fat, and of course so do biscuits, pastry and 'junk' foods. Butter, hard cheeses and red meats are high in saturated (hard) fat. Oily fish such as herring, mackerel and sardines contain polyunsaturated fats, as do vegetable oils such as sunflower, safflower and soya. A high-fat diet, especially one that includes a lot of saturated fats, raises the level of cholesterol in the blood, which is associated with a greater risk of heart disease. Cholesterol is vital in small amounts to protect the nerves and cells and produce hormones but can be harmful in large quantities. Polyunsaturated fats are thought to play a part in lowering the blood cholesterol level. A baby under two years old needs fat, and if fat were not added to milk formulas the amount of feed would have to be increased. Fat also contains fat-soluble vitamins such as vitamins A, D, E and K. Once your child is over two years old the amount of fat in the diet should be about a third of the total number of calories. However, if your child tucks in to lots of 'junk' food containing hidden fats, such as crisps, chips, beefburgers and so on, then the amount of fat in her diet will be more than she needs. Too much saturated fat can lead to clogging of the arteries, which may result in eventual heart disease in susceptible individuals.

CARBOHYDRATES

Carbohydrates – starches, sugars and fibre – are the foods that give us energy.

Natural sugars are found in fruit and vegetables, which provide many other valuable nutrients as well. However, most people think of sugar as the refined white variety that sits in the sugar bowl – this contains no protein, vitamins, minerals, fat or fibre, but only 'empty' calories. Too much refined sugar – also found in sweets, cakes, biscuits and many bought foods – is linked with tooth decay, heart disease and diabetes. A well-balanced diet without refined sugars provides all the calories your child needs. Most nutritionists recommend that we should cut our sugar intake by half. It is especially important to steer clear of added sugar when you are first weaning your baby, so that she does not develop a sweet tooth.

Starches – grains such as pasta, rice and bread, and root vegetables such as potatoes and parsnips – are complex types of carbohydrate which also contain many other vital nutrients, vitamins, minerals and proteins. Starches can be refined, i.e. stripped of these other nutrients, so that, like sugar, they provide only 'empty' calories, adding weight but not value. Convenience foods, and that includes baby foods, are often padded out with refined starch (look for the words 'modified starch' on the label), and are best used in moderation.

Fibre – commonly known as roughage – is contained in the skin and fibrous parts of fruit and vegetables, as well as in pulses, and cereals such as oats, barley and rye. We eat far less fibre than our ancestors, and this has been linked with the increase in such 'diseases of affluence' as heart disease, bowel cancer and other bowel problems. Most adults would benefit from increasing the amount of fibre in their diet by eating wholemeal bread and plenty of raw fruit and vegetables. However, caution is needed with babies and young children. Their immature digestive systems find it much harder to process foods such as pulses, and too much fibre can be one cause of 'toddler diarrhoea' and malnutrition. That does not mean that you should go to the other extreme and give your child nothing but refined carbohydrates such as squashes, jam, ice-cream and instant puddings. Such foods are full of empty calories and deprive the body of vital nutrients. The answer is to choose fresh fruit and vegetables, and good-quality carbohydrate foods. Of course, a little of what you fancy doesn't do any harm, so long as it is only eaten occasionally.

Protein

Protein is made up of amino acids, many of which can be manufactured in the body itself from foodstuffs eaten. But there is a group of amino acids called 'essential amino acids' that cannot be made in this way and have to be taken in food.

The little biology or nutrition you probably remember from school may have given you the idea that protein is only to be found in meat, fish, cheese, milk and eggs. It is true that these animal sources of protein are good sources of essential amino acids. However, today's emphasis on the importance of eating a variety of foods and steering clear of too much meat and dairy products has led nutritionists to take more notice of plant sources of protein: pulses such as beans, peas and lentils; grains such as wheat, oats and rice; and nuts and seeds. These sources of protein do not contain essential amino acids in the same proportions as animal protein but if they are combined they provide a good, healthy substitute. Traditional combinations such as baked beans on toast, rice pudding, macaroni cheese, cereal with milk, or cheese sandwiches are some examples of combined protein dishes with high food value. Protein shortages are rare in our affluent society, but children on restricted diets – such as vegans, who eat no animal protein whatsoever – have to be especially careful to eat a good mix of vegetable and cereal protein, together with appropriate supplements in order to make sure they receive the correct protein balance.

Protein is especially important for children because it is needed for growth and to repair tissues that break down. Toddlers need approximately 30 gm (1¼ oz) of protein a day – about the amount contained in five eggs, 750 ml (1½ pints) of milk, or 125 gm (4 oz) of hard cheese. If they are ill they need more protein, but as most children and adults eat more protein than they strictly need anyway, this is usually provided by their normal diet.

VITAMINS AND MINERALS

Minute amounts of vitamins and minerals are found in the food we eat and are vital to keep our bodies fit and healthy. Many vitamins and minerals work with each other – for instance vitamin D and calcium help make strong bones and teeth; Vitamin C and iron are needed for rich, well-oxygenated blood. The key to ensuring that your child gets the amount of vitamins and minerals she needs is to make sure she eats a *varied* diet which includes a lot of fresh foods. Processing food robs it of vital minerals and vitamins, which then have to be replaced artificially.

DOES MY CHILD NEED A SUPPLEMENT?

Reports that giving children a vitamin and mineral supplement can improve school performance and curb anti-social behaviour have started many parents wondering whether their children are getting enough vitamins and minerals in their diets. These results have not yet been validated and should be treated with caution. The problem is, even the experts cannot agree on the correct levels of these substances. There is also the risk of overdosing on vitamins and minerals because the body is unable to get rid of some, such as Vitamin A which is stored in the liver. Most nutritionists would argue that giving your child poor-quality food and making up any deficiencies with pills is no substitute for a proper diet. Too much fatty and sugary food will result in a shortfall of vitamins and minerals, including the vital 'nerve' vitamins and minerals (the B group vitamins, iron and zinc) that nourish the brain. The best way to ensure your child has a good-quality diet is to provide a wide variety of different foods, and then she will have all the vitamins, minerals and trace elements she needs. Only if your child is on a very restricted diet over a long period of time might she go short of essential vitamins and minerals. Even if you think your child might fit into this category it could be harmful to give her too many pills. Check with your doctor before giving her any supplements.

CALORIES

A calorie is simply a measure of energy. The calorie count of a food is the amount of heat it provides after you have eaten it. Foods contain calories in the form of protein, fat and carbohydrate. For most of us carbohydrate is the most easily metabolized, and therefore the major energy source. In a healthy diet calories come from a good range of different foods.

The number of calories needed varies according to age, sex, level of activity and so on. Children need a relatively high number of calories, because they use up a lot of energy running about and because they are actively growing. It is only if more calories are consumed than the amount of energy used that the remainder are converted to fat.

The box below gives some very rough guidelines as to how many calories your baby or toddler needs. However, counting calories for a child – unless there are special reasons to do so, for example if she is diabetic – is a pointless exercise. So long as she gets a varied diet and a minimum of 'empty calorie' foods containing too much refined sugar, starches or fat, then her appetite is the best guide to how much food she should eat.

CALCIUM

Calcium is important for strong bones and teeth, which is why children in particular need a good intake. During pregnancy and breast-feeding your baby's needs are supplied by you, so you need to take in more calcium than usual. Milk is a good source of calcium, which is why it is often recommended for young children. But if your child doesn't like milk, don't worry. There are plenty of other foods that contain calcium, such as cheese, yoghurt, cereals, sardines, pilchards and other fish with bones. There are also many ways to disguise milk – in pancakes, scones, rice pudding, custard and so on – so it is highly unlikely that your child will go short. Vitamin D – the sunshine

---

How many calories?

0 to one year	800 kilocalories a day
One to two years	1200 kilocalories a day
Two to three years	1400 kilocalories a day

Remember these are just averages, and that so long as your child seems healthy and is growing as she should, she is likely to be getting the number of calories she needs. If she is ill she may need more. If she is overweight and underactive she may need fewer.

vitamin – is vital, since without it the body cannot absorb calcium from the gut. A pre-school child needs about 600 mg of calcium a day (about the amount contained in four sardines if you leave in the bones).

Iron

Iron is vital for healthy red blood cells – the part of the blood that carries life-giving oxygen to all the organs of the body. It is also essential for healthy muscles. Some experts believe that many toddlers are short of iron. Such shortages can arise if a toddler drinks too much milk (which is a poor source of iron) and therefore has no appetite for other foods. Anaemia, or iron deficiency, can also occur if stores of iron are low at birth, for example if your baby was premature. If your child has an iron deficiency she will be pale, and the inside of her eyelids will be pale instead of pink. She will be easily exhausted, and may succumb to every passing infection. A baby needs 6 mg of iron a day, a toddler 8 mg (about the amount found in a small slice of lamb's liver). The body is able to absorb only a small amount of iron from food. It is most easily absorbed from liver, red meat and other offal, and is also found in eggs, wholemeal bread, shellfish, pulses and green vegetables (though in fact spinach, famed for its high iron content, contains an agent which blocks its absorption).

Zinc

Zinc is a trace element, and has recently hit the headlines because it is believed that many people may be suffering from a minor shortage of this mineral. Not much is known about zinc, but a highly refined diet containing too much sugar and white flour is believed to be the reason some people are short of it. Moreover, metal residues contained in certain fertilizers are believed to unbalance the amount of zinc in the body in relation to other minerals. Very high-fibre diets can create shortages because a chemical in bran prevents zinc from being absorbed. There is no recommended daily intake of zinc in this country at present, though in America an intake of 10 mg is advised for children aged between one and six. Foods rich in zinc include liver, meat, cheese, herring, shellfish, corned beef and seeds such as sunflower. It has recently been suggested that some small-for-dates babies may be so as a result of a zinc deficiency in the mother. Vegetarians who are not eating a good varied diet may also risk zinc deficiency. Ask your doctor if you or your child could benefit from a supplement.

SALT (SODIUM CHLORIDE)

Salt is important because it regulates the fluid balance in our bodies. Babies need only a minute amount of salt – the amount found in breast milk or modified formula. Too much salt is dangerous for their immature kidneys. Once your child is on solids her need for salt can be met from foods without any salt added. A shortage of salt is only likely

---

Healthy eating hints

- Cut down on fat. Cut visible fat from meat. Grill or bake rather than roast or fry.
- Watch out for hidden fat in cakes, biscuits, pastry and so on.
- Eat more polyunsaturated fats – found in oily fish, seeds and vegetable oils.
- Don't give a child under five skimmed milk, or a child under two semi-skimmed.
- Avoid sugary foods: sweets, chocolates, soft drinks, squashes.
- Check food labels to see where sugar is on the list of ingredients. If it is near the top the product is high in sugar. Watch out for sucrose, glucose, fructose – they are all forms of sugar.
- Make sure your child eats plenty of fresh fruit and vegetables.
- If there is a food your child does not especially enjoy, substitute something else (see the chart on pages 62–4 for nutrients contained in various foods).
- Don't add extra bran to your child's food.
- Avoid foods that contain 'empty calories'.
- Make sure your child has a varied diet.
- Do not give your child sweet snacks or crisps, etc., between meals, as these may spoil his appetite for more nutritious foods.
- Choose foods from each of the four basic food groups each day.
- Make sure your child spends plenty of time out of doors – to ensure an adequate supply of vitamin D, which is metabolized in the body from sunlight.
- Ensure that your child eats plenty of foods containing vitamin D (see the chart on page 82).

to occur if your child is losing salt in diarrhoea and vomiting.

Many 'junk' foods such as crisps and other salted snacks contain high amounts of salt and fat, and too much salt may lead to high blood pressure in later life in susceptible people. If there is high blood pressure in your family, it is worth making sure your child does not develop a taste for salt. Choose fresh foods; do not add extra salt during cooking, or at the table; and avoid foods high in salt such as bacon, ham, smoked kippers or haddock, packet soups and so on.

WHICH FOOD?

It is all very well knowing which nutrients are supplied by different foods, but how do you ensure that your child gets what she needs? Fortunately you do not have to memorize complicated tables of nutrients to ensure that your child gets a balanced diet. Simply make sure that each day she has a selection of food from the four basic food groups, examples of which are given below:

1. *Meat and meat substitutes*

Baked beans	Nuts
Beef	Pork
Cheese	Rabbit
Chicken	Sardines
Chick peas	Seeds
Eggs	Soya beans
Herring	Tuna
Lamb	Turkey
Liver	White fish
Mackerel	

2. *Cereals and grains*

Brown bread	Oatcakes
Crispbread	Pasta
Fruit breads	Pitta bread
Granary bread	Porridge oats and other cereals
Muesli	Rice
Muffins, crumpets, pikelets	Rye bread

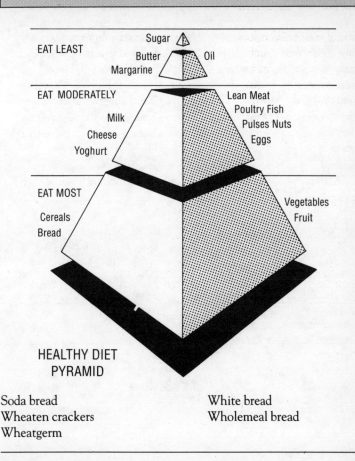

EAT LEAST

Sugar

Butter Oil

Margarine

EAT MODERATELY

Milk

Cheese

Yoghurt

Lean Meat

Poultry Fish

Pulses Nuts

Eggs

EAT MOST

Cereals

Bread

Vegetables

Fruit

HEALTHY DIET
PYRAMID

Soda bread   White bread
Wheaten crackers   Wholemeal bread
Wheatgerm

---

3. *Fruit and vegetables*

Apples	Carrots
Apricots	Celery
Avocado	Cherries
Bananas	Courgettes
Beetroot	Cucumber
Blackberries	Dried fruit
Blackcurrants, redcurrants	French beans, runner beans
Broccoli	Grapes (seedless or deseeded)
Brussels sprouts	Marrow
Cabbage	Melon

Mustard and cress
Nectarines, peaches
Oranges
Parsnip
Pears
Peas
Pineapple
Plums
Potatoes
Raspberries

Spinach
Strawberries
Swede
Sweetcorn
Tangerines, clementines
Tomatoes
Turnip
Ugli fruit, satsumas
Watercress
Watermelon

4. *Dairy foods*

Butter
Buttermilk
Cottage cheese
Cream
Curd cheese
Fromage frais

Hard cheeses e.g. Cheddar,
   Cheshire, Lancashire,
Parmesan
Whole pasteurized milk
Yoghurt

5 YOUR GROWING CHILD

Most parents gain a special sense of satisfaction from seeing their baby grow from a helpless infant into a strapping toddler. Your baby will never grow so fast as he does in his first year. By the time he is one your baby will have grown about 25 cm (10 inches) on average and will be three times heavier than he was at birth. Between the ages of one and two his growth and weight gain will slow down, and from two to three it levels to a steady rate of growth which will continue until he reaches his teens.

Remember that your child's growth rate is unique. Fascinating though it is to plot your child's progress, do not be tempted to compare him with others of the same age. Your child's individual growth and weight gain will be influenced by many factors. Birth weight is determined by your child's inheritance (whether he comes from a large- or small-built family), and by the environment in the womb. If, for example, the placenta was not working efficiently because of medical problems during pregnancy (e.g. pre-eclampsia), your baby may well be smaller than expected (i.e. small for dates). On the other hand, babies of diabetic mothers are often large. However, most babies usually catch up or slow down after birth.

The most accurate way to record your child's progress is to plot his length and weight gains on a special growth chart, like the ones kept by experts. Such 'centile' charts are extremely reliable because they are based on the growth patterns of large numbers of children of different ages, in order to take into account children who are both small and large in build.

Centile charts work like this: if, for example, your child is on the 50th centile, that means that out of 100 children of the same age, 50 would be taller and 50 would be shorter. If he is on the 90th centile 10 children would be taller than he is and 90 would be shorter. If he is on the third centile, three would be smaller and 97 would be taller.

Give or take minor fluctuations, your child should stay on the same centile. That means he is growing at the correct rate for him individually. The important thing to bear in mind is his overall progress. The health visitor or doctor will probably keep centile charts

See how your child has grown

1st year	
0–6 months	125–250 g (4–8 oz) a week
6–9 months	125 g (4 oz) a week
9–12 months	50–75 g (2–3 oz) a week
Average over the year 14 lb (6.4 kg)	
2nd year	7 lb (3.2 kg)
3rd year	5 lb (2.3 kg)

with your child's medical records, but you may like to keep your own record of your child's growth. You can use the charts on page 72 to do so. These charts show the wide range of normal weights and heights. If you have your child weighed regularly at the clinic remember that it is his progress over a period of time that counts, rather than his weekly or monthly height and weight gain. How often you choose to have your baby weighed is up to you. If you decide to have him weighed every week, you will be more aware of dips and rises in his growth than you would if you had him weighed once a month. Experts recommend that children should be weighed and measured once a month during the first year and every three to six months after that, to make sure they are progressing as they should. Some parents feel more reassured in the early weeks and months if they have their baby weighed more often than this.

HEIGHT

Like weight, height, or more accurately length, increases most rapidly during the first year. Use the chart on page 72 to assess your child's progress. Measure a baby by lying him on a flat surface against a wall. Ask someone to hold your baby's legs out straight, making sure his heels touch the wall, while you measure him. It is possible to buy attractive height charts, which can be fixed to the wall for toddlers and older children and provide a fascinating record of their growth. Get your child to stand against the wall, feet flat on the floor, looking straight ahead, then use a flat object such as a book or ruler placed on his head to mark the level of his height.

The rate at which your child grows will vary according to the season (faster in spring and summer, slower in autumn and winter), his age (fastest during the first two years, then slow and steady until adolescence), and his state of health. A bout of illness may temporarily slow down his growth, though he will usually have a growth spurt to make up for lost time once he has recovered.

You need to look at your child's growth in terms of both weight and height. He should be on the same centile for both. If he gains weight faster than he is growing in height, he may become overweight, although do bear in mind that there will be minor fluctuations. For instance, many toddlers look quite chubby before shooting up so that their weight and height are more evenly matched.

If your child has hardly grown at all over six months, measure him again after a month or so. If he still has not progressed, point this out to your doctor. Very occasionally your child's failure to grow could be due to a deficiency of growth hormones. This can now be successfully treated, so long as treatment is started early enough. However, the chances are that your child's slow growth is due to other causes, such as his genes or a spell of illness, and the doctor will be able to reassure you.

How tall will your child be when he grows up? As a rough rule of thumb, it has been discovered that on average girls are about half their adult height at eighteen months, boys at two years. Why not jot this down somewhere and see if you were right?

Growing all the time

Your child's head and brain grow rapidly during the first three years. By his first birthday the circumference of your baby's head will have grown by 12.5 cm (5 inches) – twice as much as it will grow in the next 11 years. By the time he is two, your baby's head and brain growth will be almost complete. The remaining increase in size is mostly scalp and bone. The length of your baby's body increases by 5 cm (2 inches) during the first three months; 6 cm (2½ inches) between three and six months; and 7.5–10 cm (3–4 inches) between six months and a year. Different parts of your child grow at different rates. For instance a newborn baby is top heavy: his head accounts for a quarter of the size of his body. An adult's head is about an eighth of his body. Your child's genitals, on the other hand, grow relatively slowly in the early years, speeding up once he reaches adolescence. At the age of one year your baby's head is still big compared to the rest of him. His body is chubby and pot-bellied. His legs are bowed and his feet are well padded with fat. By two years of age your child is looking less rounded. By three he is slimmer and taller, and more 'child-shaped'.

PROBLEMS OF GROWTH

Bearing in mind what has been said about individual variations in height and weight there are three questions to ask yourself if you are worried about your child's growth.

1. Is your child the appropriate build for your family? If you and his father are small-boned and short, you can expect your child to be the same.
2. Is he growing as he should? Check the growth charts on page 72 to see whether he is growing along the same centile.
3. Is his weight appropriate for his height? Your child's weight and height should be along the same centile.

OVERWEIGHT

If your child weighs at least 20 per cent more than can be expected for his age, height and build then he is overweight. It is not known for certain why some children are overweight. For years the argument has raged over whether obesity is caused by nature or nurture: that is, whether fat people inherit a tendency to gain weight because of a slow metabolism (i.e. the rate at which the body burns up food); or whether it can be blamed on eating habits. We all know people who can eat like a horse and remain skinny as a rake, while others only have to catch sight of a cream bun to pile on the pounds. One thing is certain: obesity does tend to run in families. Eight out of ten overweight children have fat parents. Fat children tend to become fat adults: one survey showed that 80 per cent of overweight teenagers grew up to be obese adults.

Some recent research carried out on babies in Cambridge throws some intriguing new light on the question. Using the latest machinery to measure energy intake and output, scientists looked at a group of babies throughout the first year. Half the babies had fat mothers and therefore could be expected to be more prone to putting on weight; half had normal-weight mothers. By the end of the first year half the babies of fat mothers had become overweight themselves. But what is revolutionary about this study is that the babies became fat not because they ate more, but because they were *less active* than the normal-weight babies. It seems that some babies are programmed by their genes to be less active, regardless of what they eat. The study proves that overeating is not the cause of fatness at this age, so relieving the guilt of some mothers who fear that they must be to blame if their children are fat. But it does not remove the responsibility. In order to avoid obesity, it is important to get the energy equation right for your child as an individual. It is much easier to prevent obesity from occurring by following the good diet rules outlined in this book than to cure it once it has occurred.

The controversy over the causes of obesity looks set to continue for many more years yet, but whatever the truth of the matter obesity is a major problem today. It is twice as common as it was 40 years ago. Overweight children are likely to be teased by their friends and to find it hard to run about and join in physical activities; overweight adults are more susceptible to a variety of illnesses in later life. These are good reasons to try and ensure that your child stays slim and fit.

Common sense will tell you if your child is becoming overweight, but you can use the growth charts on page 72 to check your suspicions, so that you can nip any potential problems in the bud. Bear in mind that children often go through temporary phases of tubbiness before a growth spurt. However, if your child is persistently too heavy for his height, take action now rather than waiting for the problem to become entrenched. It will be much easier for you to control your child's diet while he is a toddler, rather than later on when he is subject to other influences such as school, his friends and television.

The secret of keeping your child's weight under control is to ensure that he eats enough of the right nutrients without taking in too many calories which are then converted into fat. The other side of the equation is activity. Overweight people tend to be more sluggish, partly because it is harder to move around if you are carrying excess poundage.

Unless your child is seriously overweight, in which case you should seek professional advice, you should not put him on a 'diet' as such. Children are actively growing, and by restricting his intake you could be depriving him of vital nutrients. Your aim should be to keep his weight steady while his height increases. Listed below are some simple ways in which you can ensure that your child gets all the nourishment he needs without taking in extra calories; and without him noticing any difference in his diet.

● *Cut down on fats.* Spread your child's butter or margarine more thinly. Choose lean cuts of meat, and white fish rather than fatty fish. Grill, steam or braise rather than roasting or frying. There are also many healthy substitutes for high-fat products that you can use without having to resort to special diet products. For example, sorbet or low-fat frozen yoghurt instead of ice-cream; baked potato rather than chips.

- *Look out for hidden calories.* For example, tinned fruit in sugar syrup – far better to serve fresh fruit, or fruit tinned in natural juice. Cola, fizzy drinks and fruit squashes are also high in sugar and therefore calories – substitute diluted pure fruit juice or, better still, water.
- *Pay attention to the snacks your child eats.* If he eats a lot of high-calorie snacks, substitute other foods, for instance an apple instead of a bag of crisps, a pear instead of a chocolate biscuit.
- *Check your child's milk intake.* If your child drinks a lot of milk, cut down. Replace it with diluted fruit juice or with water. Ask your doctor or health visitor whether they recommend using semi-skimmed milk, but do not give skimmed milk to a child under five except on medical advice, as it may lack vital nutrients.
- *Cut out added sugar.* Don't sprinkle sugar on breakfast cereal or add it to your cooking. Your child will soon lose his taste for oversweetened foods.
- *Cut down the amount of processed food your child eats.* Readymade foods are often high in unnecessary calories. Provide freshly prepared food whenever you can.
- *Be careful when you are shopping and cooking.* If you don't buy high-calorie foods such as biscuits, cakes, sweet drinks and snacks in the first place you won't be tempted to feed them to your child. Stir fry, steam or grill rather than frying, and don't add extra fats, for example a knob of butter, to your cooking.

Born to be fat?

To a certain extent your child's propensity to be fat will depend on his basic build. Experts distinguish three major body shapes:
Ectomorph. Tall and slim, least likely to put on weight.
Mesomorph. Well proportioned and muscular, often good at sports, with a tendency to put on weight if exercise is not maintained.
Endomorph. Short with broad feet and hands. The shape most likely to have weight problems.

Your child will inherit his basic shape from his parents. Though in practice most people have elements from each of the body shapes, he will be predominantly one or the other.

- *Don't introduce solids too early.* Four to six months is soon enough for the vast majority of babies.
- *Don't force your child to finish everything on his plate.* Let him be guided by his appetite, to avoid setting up habits of overeating.
- *Don't use food as a reward or comfort.*
- *Avoid specific diet products.* It is better to accustom your child to healthy alternatives.
- *Involve the rest of the family.* You will all benefit from a healthier diet.
- *Restrict eating to one room.*
- *Encourage your child to be active.* Don't keep him confined to a pram or playpen as a baby. As he gets older provide him with activity toys such as a trike or climbing frame. Get into the habit of going for family walks. Visit the swimming pool regularly. Join Tumble-Tots – a special gymnastic organization for very young children. To find out if there is a group in your area, contact Tumble-Tots UK Ltd, Cannons Sports Club, Cousins Lane, London EC4R 3TE. Tel: 01-621 0904.
- *Don't deprive your child of the occasional high-calorie treat,* for example if he is invited out to a birthday tea. Remember it is his overall intake that is important.

Cutting the calories

The following examples of high-calorie foods with suggested low-calorie substitutes show how easy it is to reduce your child's calorie intake without keeping him short of nutrients or making him feel deprived.

High-calorie food	Low calorie alternative
10 slices tinned peaches in syrup 91 kilocals	1 medium-sized fresh peach 40 kilocals
1 small portion chips 325 kilocals	1 medium jacket potato 110 kilocals 1 apple 46 kilocals
1 small bag crisps 159 kilocals	1 low fat yoghurt with medium sliced banana 172 kilocals
1 small portion sponge pudding with custard 325 kilocals	1 fillet steamed plaice 126 kilocals
4 fried fish fingers 209 kilocals	125 g (4 oz) minced beef and chopped onion, braised 91 kilocals
1 cheeseburger 300 kilocals	

These are just a few examples. Use a calorie counter, or better still a book that gives a full nutritional breakdown of everyday foods, to help you plan your menus sensibly.

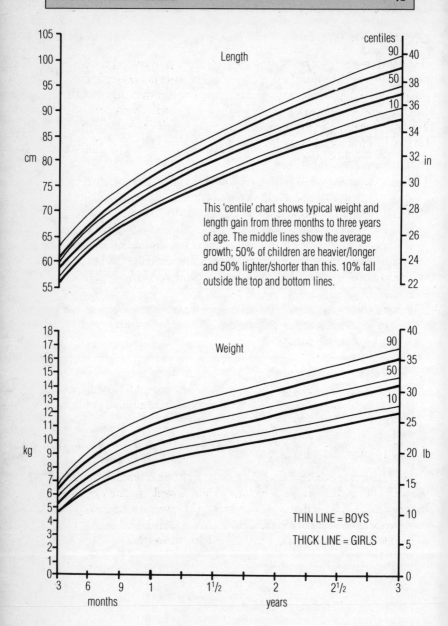

Length

centiles
90
50
10

cm in

This 'centile' chart shows typical weight and length gain from three months to three years of age. The middle lines show the average growth; 50% of children are heavier/longer and 50% lighter/shorter than this. 10% fall outside the top and bottom lines.

Weight

90
50
10

kg lb

THIN LINE = BOYS

THICK LINE = GIRLS

months years

UNDERWEIGHT

Being underweight is a far rarer problem than being overweight. In fact, given a healthy nutritious diet, few toddlers are underweight for their build, though some may be smaller and slimmer than others of the same age and sex. If you are worried, check the growth charts opposite. You will probably find that your child's weight is perfectly normal for his build. If you are anxious after checking the charts consult your doctor. There are four major causes your doctor will want to consider:

1. *Illness.* Your doctor may suggest further tests to discover whether there is a medical reason for your child's failure to grow. One in 4,000 children suffers from a shortage of growth hormone. So long as this is detected by the age of two or three it can be treated completely successfully by injections of the missing hormone and your child will grow to normal height. Other medical problems responsible for failure to thrive are coeliac disease (see page 98), in which the child is unable to tolerate gluten, a protein found in certain cereals, and cystic fibrosis, where the pancreas fails to produce enzymes necessary for digestion. In these and other rare conditions your child will need medical supervision and special dietary advice.

2. *Social reasons.* Problems such as poor, overcrowded housing conditions, lack of money and inadequate diet can all lead to failure to thrive. In this case professional support and help may be available.

3. *Inheritance.* If you, your husband and the rest of your family are all slight, your child is likely to take after you.

The chances are that your child's slow growth rate is simply a normal variation. If you keep a food diary for a couple of weeks you may be able to spot gaps in his diet that you can correct. However, if your child is born small, no amount of forcefeeding will change that, and overfeeding could lead to him being small and overweight.

6 THE VEGETARIAN CHILD

If you are vegetarian and are planning to bring up your child likewise you may be wondering how to go about it. You could also be the target of some spoken and unspoken criticism from friends, family or professionals who may fear that your child will not get enough nourishment from a diet that contains no meat. The latest research shows that vegetarian children who follow a properly balanced diet are just as strong and healthy as their meat-eating contemporaries, and may even enjoy some health advantages: a vegetarian diet tends to be low in saturated fats and sugar and high in fibre, making it just the sort of diet that is now recommended for health. On the whole, it is thought that vegetarians have lower fat levels in the blood, are less likely to become overweight, and less likely to suffer from cancer of the bowel or from osteoporosis, a brittle bone disease that affects many women after the menopause.

However, it is important to stick to a few simple rules if you are bringing up your child as a vegetarian, and not to follow cranky or faddish diets. The more limited the choice of food, the harder it is to meet nutritional needs, especially if a child who is already on a restricted diet limits her own intake by being a fussy eater. As always the keynotes are *variety* and *balance*.

If you are vegetarian you probably fall into one of two basic categories:

- Lacto-vegetarian – you include eggs, cheese, other dairy products and honey in your diet.
- Vegan – you meet your nutritional needs entirely from plant sources with no dairy foods or animal products of any kind.

Whichever type of vegetarian diet you follow it is vital that your child's diet supplies her with all her nutritional needs as well as being high in energy, since all children need food not just for body maintenance but for the growth and development of bones, teeth, organs and body tissues.

That means avoiding processed foods, which may be full of empty calories, and buying fresh food whenever possible. One potential problem for vegetarian children is meeting energy needs, and some studies have shown that vegan children are slightly shorter than other children of the same age, though still within the normal range. A diet made up of large quantities of vegetables, fruit and cereals can be bulky, so that a child with a small appetite may feel full before she has eaten enough to supply her with the right amount of energy and nutrients. To overcome this you need to ensure that everything she eats is packed with nourishment. You need to be aware of what nutrients are contained in different types of food, so that if for whatever reason your child does not eat a particular food, you can substitute another that supplies her with the same nourishment. The at-a-glance guide on page 82 and the chapter on nutritional needs will help you plan a nourishing menu.

Wholegrain cereals, nuts and seeds can be hard to chew, with the result that your child becomes bored with chewing and does not eat enough, or that nutrients are poorly absorbed because the food has not been broken down properly. Pay attention to the texture of food to make it more palatable and easier for your child to cope with. Pulses should be well cooked, mashed and puréed. Rice should be cooked in plenty of water then mixed with liquid and mashed for a baby. Nuts and seeds, important sources of many essential nutrients, should be ground into pastes. Your child is not capable of chewing whole nuts and seeds properly until she is between two and three, and an adult vegetarian diet should not be forced on a developing child.

GETTING YOUR VEGETARIAN CHILD OFF TO A GOOD START

Breast-feeding will supply your baby with all the nutrients she needs until she is four to six months old. If you cannot breast-feed, then feed your baby a suitably modified artificial baby milk based on cow's milk, or if you are vegan with a modified soya-based formula. *Do not* feed your baby grain or other pulse-based milks, or unmodified soya, cow's or goat's milk. They will not supply her with adequate nourishment and will dangerously overload her kidneys.

Vitamin B12, essential for the health of the nervous system, is not usually found in plant foods and therefore some vegans can suffer from shortages of this vitamin. Breast-fed babies rely on stores of the vitamin laid down in their livers during their time in the uterus, as well as from breast milk. In mothers suffering from a shortage of B12, stores of the vitamin may be low, with the result that their babies run the risk of B12 deficiency – signs would be irritability, lethargy, anaemia, poor feeding and loss of head control. If you are a vegan it is sensible to take a supplement of B12 during pregnancy and breast-feeding and to give your baby a vitamin B12 supplement once she starts on solids. Discuss the dose with your doctor or health visitor.

You also need to make sure that you get enough iron. Studies have shown that the iron in breast milk is especially easily absorbed. As long as you are not anaemic, breast milk should supply your baby's needs.

Breast milk contains vitamin D, but not always enough for the baby's needs, especially those with dark skins, who may need a supplement. Vitamin D is processed in the skin as a result of exposure to sunlight, so make sure your baby's skin is exposed outdoors, even if the weather is cloudy.

As a precaution against vitamin deficiencies some nutritionists

---

Food preparation and storage tips for vegetarians

- Cook grains well in plenty of water and grind to a smooth paste. By the time your baby is one year old she should be able to cope with well-cooked whole grains.
- Soak pulses overnight, drain before cooking then cover with fresh water. You should boil for 10 minutes at least and then simmer until soft. The time taken will vary depending on the type of pulse. A pressure cooker takes much of the labour out of cooking pulses. Blend and sieve them after cooking to remove the skins.
- Buy tofu fresh and store in the fridge under water. Keep it fresh by changing the water.
- Buy nuts and seeds in small amounts and use them quickly as they go off fast. Store in the fridge.
- Make nuts and seeds more digestible by soaking overnight in water and then blending to make a 'milk'. Strain to remove any pieces of whole nut.
- Boost the nutrient value of cakes, pastries and other homemade goodies by adding the following to every 250 g (8 oz) of flour: 1 tbsp soya flour; 1 tbsp dried milk; 1 tsp wheatgerm
- You can boost the nutrient value of other foods too; for example, mix egg yolk or finely grated cheese into vegetable purées.
- Don't add salt or other strong seasoning to your baby's food.
- Yeast extract is a good source of vitamin B12. Look out for a low-salt variety (available from health food stores) to avoid overloading your baby's kidneys.

advise that babies should be given vitamin drops containing vitamins A, C and D. Ask your health visitor if your baby would benefit from such a supplement.

WEANING YOUR VEGETARIAN BABY

You can introduce solids from four to six months in the same way as you would for a non-vegetarian baby. Good starter foods are banana mashed with a little breast milk or baby milk so that it is semi-liquid, apple purée, sweet potato purée, baby rice, or sieved carrot. Many

SUGGESTED FOODS FOR VEGETARIAN BABIES

Four to six months	*Six to eight months*	*Nine months to one year*
Puréed cooked apple	Finger foods – pieces	Grated carrot with
Puréed cooked	of raw apple,	peanut-butter,
carrot	carrot, rusk,	tahini or almond
Finely mashed ripe	bread, sprouted	butter
banana	beans and	Tofu
Apricot purée	sprouted seeds	Pasta with vegetable
Rice cereal	Wholegrain cereals	sauces or nut
Mashed potato	e.g. porridge or	pastes
Sweet potato purée	baby muesli	Slices of ripe avocado
	Natural yoghurt	Hummus (chick pea
	Smooth peanut	purée)
	butter	Scrambled or boiled
	Cottage cheese	egg with bread
	Chopped or sieved	soldiers
	egg yolk	Salads
	Mashed cooked	
	pulses	
	Mashed nut roast	
	Nut or seed milks	
	Nut or seed pastes	
	Fresh fruits with	
	skin removed e.g.	
	pears, peaches,	
	plums, melon	
	Cauliflower cheese	

commercial baby foods are acceptable to vegetarians. Check the label for animal products.

From about seven months, your baby can have well-cooked, mashed wholegrain cereals mixed with plenty of fluid (e.g. boiled water, breast milk or baby milk). You can also start to give your baby thick, lentil-based vegetable soups, nut creams and butters, tofu (soya curd), cottage and grated cheeses (non-animal rennet cheese is available from supermarkets and health food stores), and eggs (if eaten). Some babies are upset by pulses. Check your baby's nappies, if her motions smell sour or if she develops nappy rash after eating pulses, wait a little while before you try again. Some children cannot tolerate pulses until they are two or three years old. You can meet your child's nutritional needs with soya-based products, such as soya milk and tofu, and cereals (see the at-a-glance-guide on page 82).

Wheat is the most difficult grain to digest and is also one of the biggest culprits in causing allergies, so avoid introducing it until after your baby is six months old. Start with brown rice, thoroughly cooked and puréed to a smooth paste. If your baby tolerates this, try barley, millet, oats and maize (sweetcorn).

NUTRITIOUS COMBINATIONS

Protein foods supply your child with essential amino acids. The secret of ensuring that a vegetarian baby or child gets her full quota of essential amino acids is to combine protein foods such as grains and pulses, grains and milk foods, seeds and pulses, grains and seeds. The following are examples of nutritious food combinations:

Baked beans with wholemeal toast
Lentil soup and bread
Brown rice and lentil casserole
Rice pudding
Macaroni cheese
Cheese sandwich
Cereal and milk
Hummus (chickpea purée mixed with tahini, a sesame paste)
Peanut butter and sunflower seed spread sandwich
Wholemeal roll sprinkled with sesame seeds
Split pea soup with milk

Bread with sunflower seed spread
Scalloped potatoes (i.e. baked with cheese and milk)

Between the ages of about one year and 18 months your baby can begin
to join in family meals, though you may still need to modify the texture
of some things she eats to make them more palatable and easier to
digest.

SAMPLE MENU FOR A VEGAN BABY OR TODDLER

Breakfast
Cereal with soya milk
Wholemeal bread with dairy-free
fortified margarine and a smear of
yeast extract
Orange juice

Lunch
Puréed or mashed lentils with
vegetables, rice or pasta
Stewed fruit and custard made
with soya milk

Tea
Wholemeal bread with vegetable
pâté, nut or seed cream
Pea soup with barley
Baked apple
Soya milk

Snacks
Soya milk
Fruit

SAMPLE MENU FOR A LACTO-VEGETARIAN
BABY OR TODDLER

Breakfast
Baby muesli with grated apple, or
porridge made with milk
Wholemeal toast with butter or

margarine and yeast extract
Milk or fruit juice

Lunch
Puréed lentil casserole with rice,
potato or pasta
Peas or carrots
Milk pudding
Water or fruit juice

Tea
Wholemeal bread with cottage
cheese, grated carrot and tomato,
or scrambled egg with bread and
butter and tomato
Fruit or yoghurt
Water or fruit juice

Snacks
Milk
Wholemeal bread with nut
spread, vegetable pâté, or cream
cheese

VEGAN FACTS

If your child is brought up on a diet consisting of completely
animal-free foods, you need to take especial care that she gets enough
of the following vitamins and minerals.

VITAMIN D

This is essential for calcium absorption and the development of healthy
bones. A shortage of vitamin D can result in rickets. A British study of
vegan pre-school children revealed low intakes of vitamin D. To ensure
that your child has enough, make sure her skin gets plenty of exposure
to the sunlight. All margarines and some soya milks are fortified with
vitamin D. In addition, many experts advise a vitamin D supplement.
Ask your health visitor for advice.

VITAMIN B12

This B vitamin is vital for the healthy development and working of the nervous system. It is made by the action of certain bacteria, which are most abundant in meat, and is also found in fortified yeast extracts. In the British study mentioned above the lowest vitamin B12 intakes were found in breast-fed children. You can ensure that your child has sufficient by giving a supplement from the time she is about six months old. Include B12-fortified foods such as soya milk in your child's diet. Add fortified yeast extract to other dishes (one teaspoon a day should be enough to meet your baby's needs) from the age of 8 to 10 months.

IRON

Vital for healthy red blood cells. In the study on vegan pre-school children mentioned above, iron intake was high. However, iron is less well-absorbed from plant sources than from animal sources. Give your child plenty of iron-rich foods such as dark-green, leafy vegetables, pulses (mung beans are specially rich in iron), apricots and other dried fruit, and some seaweeds. Iron absorption is increased by vitamin C, so let your child have a cup of fresh orange juice or an orange when she has her meals. Your child can be tested for anaemia and if she is found to be short of iron, you can give her a supplement. Consult your doctor for advice.

CALCIUM

Essential for strong, healthy bones and teeth. In the British study mentioned above, calcium levels in vegan children were half the recommended daily amounts, though none of the children showed any symptoms of calcium deficiency. Calcium is found in pulses, tofu, seeds, dark-green, leafy vegetables, nuts and drinking water. In addition calcium supplements or calcium-fortified milk can be used. Ask your health visitor if your child would benefit from a supplement.

ZINC

Strengthens the immune system. It is found in whole grains, green, leafy vegetables, nuts, wheatgerm and yeast extract. A substance called phytic acid, found in spinach, parsley and bran, can hamper zinc absorption.

FOLIC ACID

Another of the B vitamins, this tends to be destroyed by the lengthy cooking needed for cereals and pulses. Ensure a good supply by including plenty of fresh vegetables in your child's diet.

AT-A-GLANCE FOOD GUIDE

This table is especially useful for vegetarians, but is also useful for mothers whose babies are going through a faddy stage. You can be sure of meeting your child's nutritional requirements if you are aware of which foods supply which nutrients and substitute the appropriate foods for the ones your child will not or cannot eat.

If you leave out	These nutrients are in short supply	Choose these foods instead
Meat, fish, poultry	Protein, iron, zinc, vitamin B12, folic acid, vitamin B1, essential fatty acids	Milk, dairy products, wholegrain cereals, pulses
Milk, dairy foods	Protein, calcium, vitamin B12, vitamin D, vitamin B2 (riboflavin)	Pulses, fortified soya milk, dark-green vegetables, nuts and seeds
Grains	Protein, iron, nicotinic acid (B vitamin), vitamin B2 (riboflavin), zinc, fibre	Pulses, dairy foods, seaweed
Pulses	Protein, iron, zinc, calcium, fibre	Grains, dairy foods
Fruits	Vitamin A, vitamin C, fibre, folic acid	Vegetables
Vegetables	Vitamin A, vitamin C, fibre, folic acid	Fruits

7 ALLERGIES AND ADDITIVES – WHY ALL THE FUSS?*

Much of the food we eat today is processed in some way. Processing is not in itself a bad thing: if some foods were not processed, food poisoning would occur. Nor is processing something new. For centuries people have smoked, pickled, salted and preserved food in sugar, alcohol, spices and herbs in order to make it edible for longer.

Food additives are simply substances that are added to food to help them keep longer, taste better, or appear more palatable. Although we tend to associate the word additive with something that is artificial, not all additives are synthesized in the laboratory. Many are naturally occurring substances such as beetroot, paprika (red pepper powder), and even some vitamins such as vitamins C and E.

However, over the last few years food additives have been criticized for causing allergies, especially in children. It is thought that some children may be especially susceptible to the effects of artificial additives because of their immature systems. Of course, not all allergies are caused by additives; many children are allergic to foods we think of as particularly natural – cow's milk, eggs and wheat, to mention three of the most common. And not all allergies are in fact true allergies; some are food intolerances (see page 87), which does not, of course, make them any less serious.

WHAT ARE E NUMBERS?

There is a lot of confusion surrounding E numbers, which were introduced on food labels in 1983. E numbers are in fact a system used by the EC to categorize those additives that are approved in EC countries. The numbers of additives start at E100 and go on into many

* Sources used in this section include *Is Your Child Allergic?* by Dr Jan Kuzemko (Thorsons), *Diets for Sick Children* by Dorothy Francis (Blackwell), *Additives: Your Complete Survival Guide* edited by Felicity Lawrence (Century), and *Additives: A Guide for Everyone* by Erik Millstone with John Abraham (Penguin).

hundreds. Not all additives have E numbers because different countries have their own rules about what is permitted. If an additive doesn't have an E number it does not necessarily mean it is suspect, simply that it has not been approved by the EC. Just to make matters even more complicated, many additives do not have numbers at all. For instance, no one knows how many flavourings are in existence, and additives that are used in processing (such as substances used to stop food sticking to the machines) do not have to be listed.

According to Maurice Hanssen, author of the bestselling *E for Additives*, there are about 400 additives, of which most have no harmful effects. However, about 80 of these are suspected of causing problems. You can find lists of these in one of the many books now available on additives. Alternatively write to: Ministry of Agriculture, Lion House, Willowburn Trading Estate, Alnwick, Northumberland NE66 2PF (England and Wales) or Scottish Home and Health Department, Foods Branch, Room 40, St Andrew's House, Edinburgh EH1 3DE (Scotland).

KNOW YOUR ADDITIVES

COLOURINGS (E100–180)

These are used to make food look more palatable or to put back colour that has leached out during processing. Some colours, such as paprika, turmeric, beetroot and caramel, have natural vegetable origins, but the majority are synthesized in the laboratory. Colourings are some of the additives most strongly incriminated in causing problems, and some of those used in the UK do not have E numbers because they are not considered safe in other countries. (In fact, the Norwegians manage without any colourings in their food at all.) In particular, according to Dr Peter Mansfield in *Additives: Your Complete Survival Guide* (Century), the azo or coal tar dyes are suspected of causing reactions in the lungs, nose, skin and eyes and of triggering hyperactivity in susceptible individuals.

PRESERVATIVES (E200–297)

Preservatives are added to foods to prevent them decomposing and so extend their shelf life. Currying, pickling and sousing have been used to preserve food for centuries. However, some of the chemical preservatives used in food are now thought to be a health risk. In particular the nitrates and nitrites (E249–252) that are used to cure meats such as bacon, ham, corned beef, hot dogs and so on, and are also used in cheeses such as Edam and in frozen pizzas, have been banned from baby foods because of the risk of blood disorders. Saltpetre (E252) can cause hyperactivity and skin and bowel problems in some allergic children. In some areas where there is a high nitrate content in the water it is advised that babies' bottles and other drinks be made up with bottled water. Your health visitor can advise you if this applies in your area.

ANTIOXIDANTS (E300–321)

These are agents which are used to prevent food going rancid when they come in contact with oxygen in the air. Unprocessed oils and fats contain nature's own antioxidant, vitamin E, but this is destroyed by processing. Vitamin C is another natural antioxidant, and is found in fruits. Oxidization is the process that occurs when an apple, pear or potato turns brown after being cut and exposed to the air.

Concern centres around two types of antioxidant: BHA and BHT (E320 and E321), and the gallates (E310–12). According to Dr Peter Mansfield in *Additives: Your Complete Survival Guide*, these have come under suspicion of causing a large number of problems, including skin irritation, wheezing, liver damage and cancer in animals. The Hyperactive Children's Group claims they also cause hyperactivity. Both these groups of additives are still being subject to safety research, and the gallates are banned from baby foods. BHA affects metabolism and is stored in body fat.

FLAVOURINGS (620–637)

These make up the largest group of additives and many are without E numbers. Though some foods, herbs and spices are used as flavourings, the majority of flavouring agents are synthesized in the laboratory. They are used to enhance flavour, to bring out flavour by stimulating the taste buds, to replace flavour lost in processing, and to add flavour to artificial foods such as jelly, instant puddings, margarine and soft drinks. Monosodium glutamate (621), which is found in soy sauce, is used to bring out the flavour of meat and savoury snacks. Research, reported in *Additives: Your Complete Survival Guide*, has shown that it can cause brain damage in newborn rats, as well as causing asthma, skin problems, hyperactivity and high blood pressure. As it can put an undue strain on babies' kidneys it should never be given to babies, and is banned from foods for young children.

Sugar (sucrose) and artificial sweeteners are also widely used as flavourings. Although officially classed as foods, because they contain calories, they have no nutritional value except to provide energy. Processed sugar has been linked with diabetes, heart disease, tooth decay and obesity. Saccharine is the oldest artificial sweetener and has often given rise to concern, as it has been found to cause bladder tumours in animals. In some countries it is banned.

Aspartame is the most controversial sweetener, found in soft drinks, yoghurt and as a sugar substitute. It has come under suspicion because some people are thought to be unable to metabolize it. Children suffering from phenylketonuria (PKU) an inherited metabolic disorder which leads to brain damage if left untreated, should avoid aspartame as it contains phenylalanine, which PKU sufferers are unable to process. For further information on the aspartame controversy, see *Additives: A Guide for Everyone*, by Erik Millstone with John Abraham (Penguin, 1988).

EMULSIFIERS, STABILIZERS, THICKENERS etc (E322–495)

These are used to bind oils and water to form an emulsion and to stop them separating out again. Some doubts have been raised about the safety of some of these additives, and their use has been limited to a certain extent. Sodium, potassium and calcium lactates (E325–7) have been implicated in liver disease, and could be especially harmful to babies and young children. A whole group of polyoxyethylenes which are made from sorbitol (432–6) have been implicated as possible causes of cancer, bowel disorders, eczema and hypersensitivity. The phosphates E450a, b and c, which are used to bulk out stews and meats, are thought to induce bowel disorders and in high doses can affect bone growth in children.

FOOD INTOLERANCE OR TRUE ALLERGY?

The word allergy is often used to describe any reaction to food.
However, a true allergy is the reaction of the body's immune system to
something that it perceives as a foreign substance, by producing high
levels of antibodies. Doctors do not fully understand the mechanism by
which allergies occur but they do agree that they are on the increase.
An allergic reaction can occur immediately after eating a particular
food or it can be delayed, occurring hours or even days after eating the
food. This type of reaction is especially hard to pin down, and is one
reason why you should introduce solid foods very gradually to your
baby's diet, leaving several days between the introduction of each new
food to make sure it does not upset your child.

The type of allergic response that occurs will depend on which part
of the body is affected. They include:

Mouth: ulcers, swollen tongue, inflammation.

Stomach and gut: colic, diarrhoea and vomiting, blood or mucus in the
motions, indigestion and wind.

Skin: swelling, eczema, rashes.

Respiratory system: nasal problems, such as symptoms of a continual
cold (rhinitis), glue ear, asthma.

Blood: anaemia.

Nervous system: migraine, hyperactivity, extreme exhaustion,
over-anxiety.

Food intolerance is when the symptoms of an allergic response

---

Foods that commonly cause reactions

Cow's milk, and sometimes goat's milk	Pork
	Nuts and nut butters
Eggs (usually the white)	Fruits e.g. tomatoes, strawberries, pineapple, oranges
Cheese	
Chocolate	Vegetables e.g. mushrooms, peas, potatoes
Wheat	
Rye	Yeast
Fish and shellfish	Spices and seasonings
Chicken	Additives
Ham and bacon	Drugs found in foods, e.g. antibiotics
Beef	Soya

Additives that commonly cause food intolerance or allergy	
Additive	*E number*
Azo dyes	
Tartrazine	E102
Sunset yellow	E110
Ponceau 4R (red)	E124
Amaranth	E123
Erythrosine (red)	E127
Benzoate derivatives	E210–19
Monosodium glutamate	621
BHT (Butylated hydroxytoluene)	E321
BHA (Butylated hydroxyanisole)	E320
Salicylate	
Sulphur dioxide	E220
Sodium nitrite	E250
Sodium nitrate	E251
Sodium metabisulphite	E223

develop without the presence of high levels of antibodies. Doctors sometimes describe this as hypersensitivity to a particular food. A specialist will be able to tell you whether your child is suffering from a true allergy or an intolerance. Do not attempt diagnosis yourself.

Finally your child may have symptoms similar to an allergic reaction if he lacks a particular enzyme necessary to digest a certain food, or if he suffers from an inherited disorder that prevents him digesting protein. For example, some babies lack the enzyme lactase which breaks down milk sugar, making them appear allergic to milk.

WHAT TO LOOK OUT FOR

If your baby or child has experienced the same symptoms several times and you suspect that he is reacting to a food, make a note of his symptoms. Try to remember occasions in the past when he has suffered the same symptoms. Many illnesses that were previously not well understood, such as three-month colic, diarrhoea, rashes and tummy upsets of various sorts, are now increasingly recognized as being allergic responses (though of course there are many other reasons why your child might experience these symptoms, so you should seek your doctor's advice). Children who come from families where there is a history of allergy are especially susceptible, so if you, your husband or any of your relatives had or have asthma, eczema, hay fever or mysterious bouts of illness which you 'grew out of', your child may suffer the same or different allergies.

The easiest way to check what your child eats is to keep a food diary for a fortnight. Record every single thing he eats, no matter how small. Once you have collected the evidence, pay a visit to your doctor, who may refer you to a specialist at the hospital. The subject of food allergy is becoming more widely accepted amongst the medical profession these days, and most areas of the UK will have a consultant paediatrician (child doctor) who has made a special study of the subject. The doctor will want to carry out a range of simple tests designed to see whether the problem is a true allergy or something else, and will advise you accordingly. Sometimes the remedy is as simple as avoiding a particular food or foods. After a period without the foods your child will probably be 'challenged' with the foods to see whether he is still allergic to them. Often it will be found that he can tolerate small amounts again without the symptoms reappearing. In fact four out of ten children with a food intolerance grow out of it within a couple of years. Occasionally, however, tolerance disappears completely and even small amounts of the foods cause illness.

A child with a tendency towards allergy or food intolerance can develop new sensitivities if his diet is not changed frequently. Finding a 'safe' diet and sticking only to that will often mean that these foods too spark off a reaction within a short time. Many allergists prefer to put children on a special rotation diet, which allows small amounts of foods regularly over a period of one to four weeks.

Cutting the amount of sugar and artificial additives your child consumes can only do good. However, if you suspect your child is allergic or sensitive to some foods you should not try to solve the problem on your own. You need skilled help to track down your child's allergies, as there is a risk that you will end up avoiding many foods needlessly, or miss foods containing something he should avoid. Furthermore, if your child needs a restricted diet you must consult a doctor or dietician, who can make sure your child's diet is properly balanced – otherwise he could become deficient in some vital nutrient.

SOME COMMON FOOD ALLERGIES AND INTOLERANCES

COW'S MILK ALLERGY

Affects one in a 100 babies, with more boys than girls being affected. Symptoms include vomiting, diarrhoea, rashes, eczema, coughs, failure to thrive, excessive crying, colic and so on. The majority of babies grow out of this by the time they are 18 months to two years old. Even babies who are breast-fed may be affected because dairy products are passed on in breast milk.

THREE-MONTH COLIC

This may be a result of cow's milk allergy in bottle- or breast-fed babies. Removing all cow's milk products from your diet for two weeks may alleviate symptoms. A bottle-fed baby will do better on a non-cow's milk formula. Don't make adjustments to your baby's feeding regime without consulting your health visitor or doctor.

TODDLER'S DIARRHOEA

Sometimes known as the 'peas and carrots syndrome', this is a condition in which otherwise healthy toddlers suffer repeated bouts of diarrhoea in which the motions contain undigested pieces of fruit and vegetables such as peas, carrots, sweetcorn and so on. No one knows quite what the reason is, and there have been many explanations, from the psychological to food intolerance. Probably the toddler finds it difficult to digest cellulose, a type of vegetable sugar. Puréeing the offending foods or removing them from the diet may help, but do not attempt to alter your child's diet in a major way without professional advice.

ALLERGIC TENSION – FATIGUE SYNDROME

Some babies and toddlers develop a condition which involves irritability and inability to relax, alternating with extreme sluggishness. There may also be other symptoms, such as aches and pains, stuffy nose and behaviour difficulties. It is sometimes the result of a delayed food allergy, and cutting out the offending foods often leads to a cure. At other times food sensitivity may be to blame. Some foods, for example strawberries, tea, coffee and soft drinks, contain chemicals that disagree with some children. Because of the difficulty of diagnosing the condition you should always seek medical advice.

HYPERACTIVITY

Continual crying, sleeplessness and an inability to settle down for even a second are all signs of hyperactivity. However, the whole subject is fraught with controversy because of the difficulty of distinguishing between the normally active baby or toddler and the one who is hyperactive. Hyperactivity often first develops between the ages of two and five, and the child may previously have experienced problems such as three-month colic and sleeping difficulties. Again, hyperactivity has kept the experts baffled. Food intolerance or allergy, especially to additives – in particular tartrazine (E102) and benzoates (E210–19) – preservatives and refined sugars are all suspected of causing problems. Some children undoubtedly show a marked improvement when put on a special diet (see below). However, as always, it is important not to attempt self-diagnosis but to seek expert advice before trying any restrictive dietary regimes.

The Feingold Diet ← To combat
An American physician, Benjamin Feingold, suggested that certain chemicals found in food were responsible for hyperactivity. In particular, a group of chemicals called salicylates, found in almonds, apples, tomatoes, many other fruits and vegetables (see below), and aspirin, came under suspicion, as did colourings derived from coal tar or azo dyes. He devised a special additive-free diet, which he claimed resulted in a massive improvement. However, subsequent studies have failed to confirm Feingold's good results, and while it is recognized that some hyperactive children do get better on the diet the most recent study has concluded that the diet 'should not be universally applied'. It has been suggested that one reason some hyperactive children appear to improve on the diet is because of the increased attention they get and the changes in family interaction that take place as a result of their problem being taken seriously. It has also been pointed out that the diet may be harmful in the long run by causing the child to feel different, or

---

Food avoided in the Feingold diet

Almonds, apples, apricots, blackberries, cherries, currants, grapes, raisins, nectarines, oranges, peaches, plums, prunes, raspberries, strawberries
Margarine, ice-cream, cereals, sweets, gum, frankfurters, jam, tea, soft drinks
In addition, aspirin-based medicines (these should not be given to children under 12 anyway), toothpaste, mouth washes, perfumes and mint-flavoured products are excluded.

---

that he is being punished by not being allowed to eat the same as other children. If you do decide to try the diet you should do so only under medical supervision to make sure your child receives sufficient nutrients. Putting the rest of the family on the diet will help your child feel less the odd one out. If there is an improvement in his condition after four to six weeks he may be put on a modified version of the diet.

URTICARIA (nettle rash)

Food allergy or sensitivity is a well-recognized cause of urticaria, and symptoms can often be dramatic. Foods commonly causing reactions include milk, egg, nuts, shellfish, cheese, wheat, strawberries and many others. Azo dyes, benzoate derivatives, and other preservatives and antioxidants are often involved.

ASTHMA AND RHINITIS

There has been little research so far into food as a cause of asthma and rhinitis, which is like having a continual cold. Milk, eggs, the azo dyes, wheat and other cereals have all come under suspicion of causing attacks. But precise diagnosis and treatment is difficult because of delayed reactions and because other factors such as exercise, temperature and so on may be involved.

ECZEMA

About five per cent of children experience eczema at some time, often in babyhood. Other factors are often involved such as house dust, mites, animal fur, pollens and so on. But food intolerance is common and several studies have shown that many children improve on a diet that eliminates certain foods such as milk, egg, beef and chicken. Again artificial colourings and preservatives, especially the azo dyes and benzoate derivatives, have been found to make symptoms worse.

CONCLUSION

If reading this chapter has made you depressed, do bear in mind that problems with food allergy and intolerance are often only temporary and that many children grow out of them with or without treatment. If your child does suffer a food allergy, keep in touch with your medical advisers. They will probably want to review any special diets and treatment every year or so to check on nutritional balance, plus practical aspects such as holiday catering hints, what to do when your child starts school, goes to a party and so on.

How to prevent allergies developing

With the best will in the world you will not be able to prevent all allergies developing. However, there are one or two measures you can take to give your child the best chance of avoiding them.

- Breast-feed if you can for as long as possible. Avoid giving top-up bottles of cow's milk, fruit juices and so on in the early months.
- If you suffer food intolerances and are breast-feeding, avoid commonly provoking allergens such as milk, eggs and foods you know you are allergic to.
- Pay close attention to your own diet. Make sure you eat enough foods containing calcium, folic acid, riboflavin and iron.
- If you cannot breast-feed, use a modified cow's milk formula, unless your health visitor or doctor suggests you try a non-cow's milk one.
- Avoid giving solids for at least four to six months, starting later rather than earlier so long as your baby is thriving on milk alone. Avoid commonly sensitizing foods such as milk, eggs, wheat, nuts, shellfish, citrus and berry fruits for at least six months, and possibly for over a year if you or your husband are allergic to these foods.

---

8 SPECIAL NEEDS

PREMATURE BABY

If you have given birth to a premature baby you are bound to be worried and anxious. The staff in the special care baby unit will encourage you to play as full a part as possible in caring for your baby, and there will probably be somewhere you can stay in the hospital to be near your baby.

Premature babies need particularly careful feeding in order to enable them to catch up on their growth. Helping with your baby's feeds, and providing breast milk (if you are intending to breast-feed your baby) are some of the positive things you can do to help her.

The sucking reflex doesn't develop until 32 to 34 weeks of gestation, so if your baby was born earlier than that she will usually be fed by means of a fine plastic tube which is passed down her nose and into her stomach. You will probably be able to give your baby some or all of her tube feeds. The staff will show you how to hold her so that she gets the most out of her feeds. Your baby may be fed with breast-milk expressed by you or, if the hospital has one, from a milk bank, or with a special pre-term baby milk. If you are expressing your own milk, it may have to be supplemented with extra nutrients or a pre-term baby milk. The breast milk produced by mothers of pre-term babies differs in composition from that produced by a full-term mother: it is higher in protein and minerals, making it specially suitable for a premature baby. In addition, breast milk's anti-infective properties make it especially valuable in helping a pre-term baby fight off infections to which she is prey because of her shaky start in life.

The staff on the unit will show you how to express your milk using an electric or hand pump; if you have to go home and leave your baby in hospital for a while, you may be able to take an electric pump home with you, or hire one so you are able to keep up your milk supply. You will need to pump off milk regularly – every three hours – in order to keep up a good supply. Although it is difficult advice to follow, keeping a relaxed and positive frame of mind will help your milk supply. If

How to use an electric breast pump

1. Pump at least four or five times a day to help build up your supply and relieve painful engorgement (swelling).
2. Start pumping as soon after birth as you can. Your baby will benefit from the special high-antibody colostrum which is produced before the milk proper.
3. Don't worry if you do not appear to be producing a lot of milk; premature babies only need small quantities at first.
4. When pumping, make yourself comfortable. Put a plastic shell over your other nipple to catch any drips, and have a drink beside you as you will probably feel thirsty.
5. Relax by practising deep breathing or listening to some soothing music. Think of your baby as you pump. Pump for about five minutes on one side then change over to the other breast to produce the most milk possible.
6. To increase your supply, pump more frequently for a couple of days.

your baby is very tiny and/or ill she may be too weak even to be fed by tube. In this case she will be given a special 'cocktail' of nutrients intravenously.

As your baby gets stronger she will be able to start sucking from the breast or bottle. The staff will show you how to hold your baby and encourage her to suck. At first she will still be weak, and her sucking may not be sufficient to stimulate your supply if you are breast-feeding. In this case you will probably need to continue pumping or expressing in order to maintain the quantity of milk you are producing. As your baby becomes bigger and stronger she will gradually begin to take all her feeds from the breast or bottle. Once your baby's condition is stable and she is feeding well you will be able to take her home. You will probably be able to stay on the unit with your baby for a couple of days first until you have gained some confidence in caring for her.

Breast-feeding a premature baby can bring a special sense of satisfaction, but it is not always easy. The staff on the unit will help and encourage you. It is also worthwhile contacting one of the breast-feeding organizations, who have a lot of experience in helping mothers in this situation and who will probably be able to put you in touch with another mother who has breast-fed a premature baby.

FEEDING A SICK CHILD

If your child is ill she will probably lose her appetite. It is better to give her frequent, light snacks during her illness rather than try and force her to eat 'proper' meals. She needs plenty of fluids, especially if she is running a temperature, in order to replace moisture lost in sweating, or if she has diarrhoea and is vomiting. Small, frequent drinks will go down better than large glasses or cups. It doesn't matter what she drinks. Your child may find fizzy drinks more palatable than still ones when she is ill.

Good nutrition is especially important to help your child fight off and recover from infection. Offer her nutritious, easily digestible foods, such as eggs, fish, and soups.

Tips on feeding your sick child

- Jellies, blancmange, junket, custards all slip down easily and are light and easily digestible. You could fortify jellies by adding whipped evaporated milk.
- Scrambled egg, mashed banana, macaroni cheese and soups are all light and easy to digest. Soft foods are especially suitable if your child has a sore throat or an illness such as mumps.
- Drinks are a way of boosting nourishment if your child is off her food. Offer her milk, milk shakes and savoury drinks.
- If your child is reluctant to drink, tempt her by putting her drink in a special beaker or giving her a curly straw. Try dipping the top of an unbreakable glass in egg white then in caster sugar to give a frosted effect. Decorate the drink with a cocktail stick with a cherry or a slice of orange or pineapple. Add a cocktail umbrella or stirrer.
- Fruit ice cubes and ice lollies go down well, especially if your child has a sore throat. Alternatively buy some of the special, fancy shapes you can freeze and put in drinks to cool them.
- Fizzy drinks can be made by adding carbonated spring water to fruit juice.
- If your child is on antibiotics give her yoghurt. Antibiotics kill off both 'bad' and 'good' bacteria in the gut. Yoghurt can help restore the balance.
- A baby who has been weaned may want to go back to the breast or bottle temporarily. A toddler who has been drinking from a proper cup may find it easier to drink from a trainer beaker again until she is better.
- As your child gets better her appetite will return. Gradually reintroduce her usual diet, being guided by your child's appetite as to how fast you do so.

DIETS FOR MEDICAL CONDITIONS

If your child has a medical condition that requires a special diet, you will need to keep in close contact with your doctor and dietician. This section gives some very broad guidelines for parents with children suffering from two such conditions, diabetes and coeliac disease. It is beyond the scope of this book to give any more than these brief outlines. For further information, contact the societies mentioned below.

DIABETES

Diabetes results from a shortage of insulin, a hormone released by the pancreas gland, which enables the body to digest sugar. Diabetes is fairly rare in babies and very young children, and can be extremely hard

---

TRAFFIC LIGHT SYSTEM OF FOOD CHOICES

GREEN (GO)   Foods that should make up a regular part of the diet
Wholemeal bread and cereals, fruit, vegetables, lean meat, fish, low-fat spreads, cheese, skimmed milk.

AMBER (CAUTION)   Foods that should be used with care
White bread, pastries and pies, fatty meat, pâté, butter, nuts.

RED (STOP)   Foods that are to be avoided except in special circumstances e.g. hypoglycaemia (low-blood-sugar episodes)
Sugar, glucose, sugary foods, sweets, chocolate, iced cakes, prepared puddings, sweetened desserts.

You can still use bought baby foods and convenience foods if you wish. Obtain a carbohydrate and calorie counter such as *Countdown*, produced by The British Diabetic Association, who will also be able to give you a wealth of information and support in caring for your diabetic child. Write to The British Diabetic Association, 10 Queen Anne Street, London W1M 0BD

---

to diagnose, since symptoms such as increased thirst and increased urination may be masked. You will need to work closely with your child's medical advisers, who will devise a diet designed to keep her blood sugar level in the correct balance.

Today's diabetic diet is extremely similar to the sort of diet recommended elsewhere in this book for health – namely high-fibre, low-sugar, low-fat. So your diabetic child will probably be able to eat much the same as the rest of the family, with perhaps a few minor adaptations. Your child's needs will be changing rapidly at this stage, and regular consultations with the dietician will be necessary to make sure these needs are met by her diet.

Certain modifications to the sort of diet followed by older children and adult diabetics are advised for babies. For instance, it is not recommended that babies and children under five have skimmed milk. Although fibre is important it is also essential that your child does not eat so much bulky food that it reduces her appetite for other things. Your child will need to eat regularly, and between-meal snacks are an important part of her regime. The dietician will probably suggest foods such as dried fruit, which are nourishing and supply her with the calories she needs.

There is no need for your child to miss out on parties and other social occasions. She can even have small amounts of treats such as jelly and ice-cream so that she does not feel different from other children. Once your child starts playgroup, you will need to inform the supervisor about her condition and her need for regular nourishment.

COELIAC DISEASE

Coeliac disease is a wasting illness in which the body is unable to digest gluten, a type of protein found in wheat and rye. Gluten damages the bowel, leading to poor absorption. Removing gluten from the diet allows the bowel to return to normal so that normal absorption occurs. Symptoms of coeliac disease are irritability, lethargy and weight loss. Your child will have a swollen abdomen, poor appetite, and pale, bulky, frothy, foul-smelling bowel motions that are difficult to flush down the toilet because they contain a lot of fat.

If your child is diagnosed as suffering from the disease she will have to stay on a gluten-free diet for life. Your doctor or dietician will advise you on what foods your child can safely eat.

Manufactured food containing gluten

(Check by brand in the list of gluten-free products produced by the Coeliac
Society). Also check labels for ingredients such as flour, cereal binder,
wheat starch, rusk, edible starch and so on.
Baby foods, including cereals, dinners and desserts
Sausages, beefburgers, tinned meat, hamburgers
Fish fingers, cod bites
Coatings used on fish or meat
Thick soups, gravy, gravy mixes, some spices and herbs
Flavoured crisps
Ready-to-eat meals and takeaways
Sauces and ketchups
Tinned vegetables in sauce, e.g. baked beans, vegetable salad
Pie fillings, some brands of fruit or fruit-flavoured yoghurt
Some sweets and coated chocolates such as Smarties
Ice-cream, mousses

If your child suffers from coeliac disease you will need to be an
especially careful label watcher, as many processed foods are thickened
with wheat starch. The Coeliac Society can supply you with lists of
manufactured foods that are free from gluten, and help you learn what
to look out for. Some manufacturers have taken to labelling food with
the crossed wheat symbol to indicate that they are gluten-free. You will
soon learn the cooking techniques necessary to make gluten-free food
attractive and palatable.

When your child is first diagnosed as having coeliac disease you will
be advised what foods she can eat, and the dietician will probably
suggest a vitamin and mineral supplement to deal with any nutritional
deficiencies. You should teach your child as soon as possible that
certain foods upset her, but at the same time try to help her live a
normal life and not feel 'different'.

Tips on providing a gluten-free diet
- Try to provide the same food for all the family so your child does not
  feel the odd one out.
- Thicken stews, casseroles, custards and so on with cornflour.
- Use gluten-free substitutes for home-cooked dishes such as pasta.
- Store gluten-free alternatives in the freezer for convenience.
- Slice gluten-free bread and keep it in the freezer to be used as
  required.

- Gluten-free hamburgers can be made with mince, and some butchers will make up gluten-free sausages.
- Suitable puddings include fruit, cheese and gluten-free biscuits, or gluten-free ice-cream or yoghurt.
- If your child is invited to a party the hostess will need some menu suggestions. Encourage your child to take along some gluten-free bread, biscuits or cake to share with the others.

Suggested day's meals for a coeliac baby

Breakfast   Milk
Baby rice mixed with milk
Lunch   Minced meat, fish or chicken with gluten-free gravy thickened with cornflour; boiled potato or mashed potato; puréed vegetables
Fruit purée
Snack   Gluten-free bread or biscuit, fruit juice
Tea   Custard or ground rice made with milk and gluten-free custard powder, and/or fruit purée
Gluten-free bread and margarine or gluten-free bought baby food

---

For further information and support write to The Coeliac Society, PO Box 220, High Wycombe, Bucks, HP11 2HY.

9 BUYING AND STORING FOOD

The food you buy depends on your tastes, how much time you have, cost and availability. If you have small children their tastes will also affect what you buy, and faddy eaters have considerable power over the meal table. The increase in the number of families where both parents work, plus the greater availability of convenience foods, has meant that family meal times are no longer the sit-down affairs they once were, and the person who prepares the food may well find him or herself preparing a different meal for each member of the family instead of one big one.

SHOPPING TIPS

FRUIT AND VEGETABLES

- Experts recommend that we should all eat more fruit and vegetables. Fruit provides natural sweetness and makes a suitable dessert for every member of the family. It can help prevent acquiring a taste for foods with added sugar. Organically grown fruit and vegetables are produced without using chemicals and are becoming more widely available.
- Take advantage of any food markets, but only choose high-quality vegetables and fruit.
- Choose vegetables that look and feel fresh. Avoid any that look old, wilted or blemished.
- Buy vegetables such as potatoes in bulk from a reputable supplier. If you live near the country it is often possible to obtain them direct from the farmer.
- Fruit should be firm and glossy. Avoid any that look old or wrinkled or that are squashy or bruised. Buy soft fruit such as strawberries and raspberries on the day you plan to eat them.
- Avoid handling fruit and vegetables too much as this can damage them.

DAIRY FOODS

- If you have milk delivered, bring it in as soon as possible after delivery, as leaving it standing on the doorstep destroys some of its nutrients.
- When buying eggs look at the date stamp to ensure they are fresh. To check an egg at home, put it in water: if it is stale it will float, if it is fresh it will sink. A fresh egg has a firm, plump yolk, and transparent, jelly-like white. A stale egg has a flat yolk and watery, spreading white, and may smell. Eggs can be a source of the food-poisoning bacteria, salmonella. Free-range eggs are a wiser choice as the birds are reared in healthier conditions. Most supermarkets now stock them.
- Buy cheese that looks and smells fresh. Avoid any that appears mouldy or overripe. Do not give too many processed cheeses, spreads and Dutch cheeses to small children because they contain a lot of additives.
- If you use butter choose the unsalted variety. Buy the sort that is wrapped in foil, as riboflavin (one of the nutrients in butter) is destroyed by light.

MEAT

- Buy lean meat that is a good colour (dark-red beef, pale-pink pork, pinkish-red lamb) and without too much visible fat. Free-range poultry is now available in many butchers' and supermarkets and generally has a better flavour than the battery-reared variety.
- Poultry should look firm and shiny. Avoid any that appears bruised.
- Buy liver and other forms of offal on the day you intend to eat it (unless you are planning to freeze it). Choose liver that looks bright and shiny and smells fresh.
- Avoid smoked and cured meat products for babies and toddlers.
- Meat pies and other made-up meat products such as beefburgers and sausages often contain a lot of hidden fat and ingredients such as cereal, which make them unsuitable for babies and small children. Make your own, using good ingredients.

FISH

- Whole fish should have firm flesh, clear shiny eyes, red gills and smell clean. Steaks and fillets should have firm, dense flakes. If the fish looks watery or has a greenish or bluish tinge it is a sign it is not fresh.
- Avoid smoked and cured fish and shellfish for children, as the former contain many suspect additives, and the latter are one of the biggest culprits in sparking off allergies.
- Always buy fish on the day you intend to eat it (unless you plan to freeze it on the day of purchase).

STORAGE

FRUIT AND VEGETABLES

- Store in a cool place such as a pantry, if you are lucky enough to have one, or the refrigerator (except for bananas)
- Fruit and vegetables such as apples, soft fruits, sprouts, broccoli, cabbage, lettuce, mushrooms, peas, watercress and so on keep best if stored in a polythene bag. Aubergines, courgettes, citrus fruits, peppers and tomatoes may be stored unwrapped.
- Potatoes and other root vegetables should be kept in a cool, dark place.
- Fruit that you are trying to ripen, such as bananas or pears, should be kept at room temperature.

DAIRY FOODS

- Store milk in the refrigerator.
- Eggs will keep longer if you store them in a covered container in the refrigerator. They will stay fresh for two to three weeks. Store away from strong-smelling foods, as their smell may contaminate the eggs.
- Wrap cheese in cling film or greaseproof paper and store in a cool place. Do not keep mouldy cheese.
- Store butter in the refrigerator covered to avoid light destroying its vitamins.
- Buy soft cheeses in small quantities and use quickly, as they do not keep well.

MEAT AND FISH

- Meat and poultry will keep for three days in the refrigerator. Never let raw meat come into contact with cooked meat as it could cause bacterial contamination.
- Before cooking frozen chicken defrost it completely, otherwise bacteria could contaminate it if it is not well cooked.
- Offal should be eaten on the day you buy it. If it is frozen, you can keep it in the freezer for up to a month.
- Fish is best eaten within 12 hours of buying it.

OTHER STORAGE HINTS

- Never store food in a tin once it has been opened.
- Throw away mouldy foods, as the mould may have penetrated the whole item even if you cut the mouldy bits off.
- Never refreeze frozen fish or meat.
- Do not leave food uncovered in hot weather even for a moment, or it could be contaminated by flies.
- Always cover and refrigerate any leftovers as soon as they have cooled down.
- Do not put hot food straight into the fridge as it will cause an overall rise in temperature which could start bacterial action in foods stored in there.
- Take care to reheat any cooked foods thoroughly.
- Do not buy or eat foods that are past their 'sell-by' date.
- If you buy frozen food, put it in your freezer within an hour of purchase to avoid partial thawing.
- Do not keep cooked food for more than two days.
- Check that your fridge and freezer are the correct temperature. Freezers should be between $-0.4°F$ ($-18°C$) and $-9.4°F$ ($-23°C$). Use a fridge thermometer to ensure your fridge is cold enough. It should be between $34°F$ ($1°C$) and $39°F$ ($4°C$).

FOOD POISONING

At the time of writing, food poisoning never seems to be far from the headlines. The recent wave of food-poisoning epidemics, such as salmonella and listeria, has been partly caused by the revolution in food-production techniques and the changes in our patterns of buying, cooking and eating food.

Many more of us today buy ready meals, takeaways and meals in restaurants than we did a few years ago. Intensive rearing of poultry for eggs and meat, plus the increase in sales of processed meat which can become contaminated during processing, have both added to the problem. The trend towards fewer additives, admirable though it is, has led to food going off more quickly. This means that it is extra important to observe strict hygiene rules in the kitchen.

The culprits

- *Cook-chill meals*   Ready-made recipe meals are not cooked thoroughly enough beforehand to kill off all bacteria. That means it is especially important to cook them thoroughly at home. Always follow the packet instructions to the letter, and also observe the manufacturer's instructions if you are reheating in a microwave, to avoid 'cool spots' where the food has not been cooked through.
- *Prepacked salads*   These look clean, so many people don't bother to wash them. Always wash carefully under running water.
- *Ready-made sandwiches*   Keep them in a fridge and eat them the same day. Avoid those on display unwrapped, for example in a pub or sandwich shop.
- *Eggs*   Always cook thoroughly. Boil for seven minutes and cook omelettes and scrambled eggs until all the runny bits have been eliminated. Free-range eggs from a reliable source are a safer buy than eggs from battery farms.
- *Poultry*   Buy from a reputable supplier. Cook carefully and do not stuff, as this prevents heat reaching the centre of the meat. Instead cook the stuffing separately in a covered container.
- *Processed meat, sausages, mince, hamburgers*   Cook thoroughly. Bacteria can be spread through the product during processing.
- *Soft cheeses, such as Brie, Camembert and goat's cheese, and unpasteurized dairy products*   Avoid giving them to children under three, and avoid them yourself if you are pregnant.

WATCH THAT LABEL

By law, most prepacked foods have to carry a list of ingredients. However, some sweets and chocolate, dairy foods, fresh fruit and vegetables, alcoholic drinks, vinegar and carbonated water do not come under the regulations.

Ingredients are listed in descending order of weight. Added water is not listed unless it constitutes more than five per cent of the weight of the finished product. However, that isn't the whole story. It is not always possible to see what the main ingredient is because there are ways of disguising it. For instance, sugar may be the main ingredient in a product, but the manufacturer may have used different types of sugar such as corn syrup, fructose (fruit sugar), lactose, and so on, which added together constitute quite a lot of sugar but individually come fairly low down on the list of ingredients.

Food additives are listed by name and E number, where one exists, with the exceptions of flavourings, modified starches and enzymes, which are listed by their descriptive name only. Furthermore, many flavourings do not have a number, and it is unknown just how many there are (estimates suggest over 3,500). Additives classed as processing aids, such as solvents, bleaches and so on, are not listed either.

Foods also contain a sell-by date or best-before label, which will usually show the date by which you should eat it. You need to read labels very carefully to be sure of what you are getting. For instance, a raspberry-flavour yoghurt does not contain any raspberries; a raspberry-*flavoured* one has had a brush with a raspberry, while a raspberry yoghurt is made with real raspberries. Confusing, isn't it?

The phrase 'free from artificial flavourings, colourings and preservatives' is not as simple as it seems at first sight either. Flavourings that have been made in the laboratory but have the same chemical make-up as natural ones count as natural. And additives that do not fall into the category of flavouring, colouring or preservative may also be contained in products labelled like this, so make sure you read the detailed list of ingredients before you buy.

These days manufacturers are responding increasingly to public pressure for healthier food. However, there is still a long way to go. Many processed foods avoid one problem only to fall into another. Thus something labelled as low fat may be high in sugar, and so on. So whenever you buy a manufactured product study the label thoroughly for information that is not contained in the publicity.

10 RECIPES

The following recipes are suitable for babies from six months unless otherwise stated. Recipes suitable for vegans are marked with an asterisk.

First tastes

Chicken casserole
1 small, boneless chicken breast
1 stalk celery
1 medium potato, peeled and quartered
1 large carrot, peeled and sliced
1 small tin tomatoes
1 small slice swede or turnip, chopped
pinch of dried mixed herbs

Put all the ingredients into a small casserole and top up with a little water. Cover with a tight-fitting lid and cook in a moderate oven for about 1 hour, or until the chicken and vegetables are cooked. Remove the chicken, chop and mince finely in a blender or food processor. Drain the liquid from the vegetables and reserve. Mash or process the vegetables to the required texture and stir in the chicken, moistening with a drop or so of cooking liquid. Reheat thoroughly when required or freeze.

For babies over eight months, add a little chopped onion. For babies over one year flavour the casserole with a little yeast extract (stock cubes are too strongly flavoured).

Quick steak dinner
Brush a 75 g (3 oz) piece of rump steak with a tiny drop of vegetable oil and grill until the juices run clear. Pat between layers of kitchen paper to remove any grease. Trim off any fat or gristle and chop finely. Process until well minced and mix with 175–200 g (6–7 oz) mashed cooked vegetables. Carrot, potato, greens and cauliflower are all

suitable. Moisten with a drop of water or some juice from a can of tomatoes. For older babies you can add a little yeast extract for extra flavour. Reheat thoroughly when required or freeze in small containers – yoghurt pots wrapped in foil and labelled are ideal.

Fish pie
2 small white fish fillets (cod, haddock, whiting, plaice), skinned
1 tinned tomato
4 tbsps milk, boiled then cooled
1 tbsp chopped parsley
wholewheat breadcrumbs

Steam the fish on a covered plate over a pan of simmering water until the flakes separate easily. Check thoroughly for any bones. Mash with the tomato, milk and parsley. Bind with enough breadcrumbs to give a suitable consistency. Reheat thoroughly as required or freeze.

Vegetarian alternative   Mix mild grated cheese with the remaining ingredients instead of fish.

Oily fish such as mackerel, herring and so on are nutritious, but not as easily digested as white fish. Delay introducing until your baby is over one year old. Tuna is an oily fish, but if you buy it canned in brine rather than oil and use it sparingly it is suitable for babies from 9 or 10 months onward.

FOR VEGETARIAN BABIES

Cauliflower cheese
6 cauliflower florets
2 small potatoes, scrubbed and quartered
50 g (2 oz) low-fat cream cheese
1 tbsp chopped parsley

Simmer the cauliflower and potato in a covered pan until tender, drain then mash with the cheese and parsley, adding a drop of milk if the mixture is too thick. Reheat when required or freeze.

Vegetarian medley
2 tbsps brown rice
2 tbsps split red lentils

1 stick celery, washed and chopped
2 carrots, peeled and chopped
2 hardboiled egg yolks
1 tbsp chopped parsley

Put the rice in a small pan and just cover with water. Bring to the boil
and simmer for 10 minutes then add the lentils, celery, carrots and a
drop more boiling water. Simmer for a further 25 minutes, drain and
reserve the liquid. Process briefly with the egg yolks and parsley, adding
a drop of the cooking liquid if necessary. Reheat as required or freeze.
As your baby grows older, try adding a little yeast extract and tomato
purée for extra flavour. A little grated cheese can add extra
nourishment too.

FAMILY MEALS

The sooner your baby can start eating meals with the rest of the family
the easier it will be for you. The following are all family recipes which
can be adapted for babies from six months onwards. The recipes serve
four people, including several portions for the baby. They can be made
up without seasoning, which can then be added once you have
removed the baby's portion or at the table.

Liver with fresh orange (suitable, if puréed or mashed, for babies
from six months)
4 tbsps corn oil
1 orange, sliced
450–500 g (¾–1 lb) lamb's liver, trimmed and thinly sliced
3 tbsps wholemeal flour
1 large onion, peeled and chopped
1 clove garlic, crushed (optional)
300 ml (½ pint) stock (not made from a stock cube for a baby)
grated rind and juice of 1 orange
½ tsp dried herbs
2 tbsps chopped parsley

Heat the oil in a pan and fry the orange slices for a minute or so.
Transfer to a serving dish and keep warm. Toss the slices of liver in the

flour. Add the onion and garlic to the pan and cook for 5 minutes. Add the liver and fry until brown but tender, then transfer to a warm serving dish. Stir in the stock, orange rind and juice, and herbs. Cook rapidly for a few minutes, uncovered, and then pour over the liver. Garnish with the orange slices, sprinkle with the parsley and serve with brown rice and a green vegetable.

Lamb and bean pot (suitable, if mashed, for babies from nine months)
125 g (4 oz) dried haricot beans
2 tbsps oil
1 kg (2 lb) boned neck lamb, cubed
2 cloves garlic, crushed
300 ml (½ pint) stock (not made from stock cube for a baby)
400 g (14 oz) can tomatoes, chopped
8 button onions
2 large carrots, peeled and sliced
1 tsp dried rosemary
2 bay leaves

Soak the beans overnight. Rinse, cover with fresh water, bring to the boil and simmer until nearly tender. Heat the oil in a pan, brown the meat in it and transfer to an ovenproof casserole. Add the garlic to the pan, fry briefly, then swill out with the stock and add to the casserole with the tomatoes, onions, beans, carrots, rosemary and bay leaves. Cover and cook in a slow oven for 1½–2 hours or until the meat is tender. Suitable for freezing.

Golden lentil soup
175 g (6 oz) split red lentils, washed
1 stick celery, washed and chopped
2 large carrots, peeled and chopped
1 small onion, peeled and chopped
2 bay leaves
900 ml (1½ pints) homemade stock or water
2 tsps lemon juice
2 tbsps chopped parsley

Put all the ingredients except the lemon juice and the parsley into a pan and simmer for 25–30 minutes. Remove the bay leaves. Liquidize

until smooth and stir in the lemon juice and parsley, adding more liquid
if the soup is too thick. For a main meal, serve with jacket potatoes or
wholemeal bread and cheese. For the baby, mash the bread or potato
into the soup for easier feeding. Suitable for freezing.

Fish cakes

You need equal quantities of unsalted mashed potato and steamed
white fish such as cod or haddock. Flake the fish and check carefully for
bones. Mash the fish and potato together and add plenty of chopped
parsley for flavour. Bind with egg yolk – or whole egg for babies over
eight months. Form the mixture into cakes, small ones for the baby,
using damp hands. Roll the cakes in wholewheat breadcrumbs or
wholewheat flour and open freeze on trays. When firm, pack into rigid
containers. Thaw in the refrigerator before cooking. Fry in hot oil or
grill, and serve with tomatoes and peas. For a baby it is best to bake or
grill a fish cake and mash some tomato into it for easier feeding.

Roast chicken dinner

Put a bunch of fresh herbs in the cavity of a chicken for flavour then
roast it without adding any seasoning or fat. To make a giblet gravy put
the giblets into a pan with 1 bay leaf, 1 chopped celery stick, 1 scrubbed
and chopped carrot, some parsley stalks and ½ small peeled onion.
Cover with water and simmer for 25 minutes. Strain and skim off any
fat with a spoon. You can add the juices from the roasting tin but skim
off any residual grease first. If you prefer a slightly thickened gravy, add
a little cornflour mixed to a paste with a drop of cold water.

Serve the chicken with plain jacket potatoes and two other fresh
seasonal vegetables. Put the required portion of chicken and vegetables
for the baby through a food mill or food processor but do not
overprocess. Moisten with gravy. From the age of six months onwards
your baby will enjoy a little more texture. Try mincing the meat and
mashing the vegetables. You can give your baby a roast meat dinner
using beef. To make gravy, use a good homemade stock (no stock
cubes) and the roasting juices with the fat skimmed off.

Chicken and bean pot

4 boneless chicken breasts, skinned
1 stalk celery, washed and chopped
400 g (14 oz) can tomatoes

1 small onion, peeled and chopped
1 large carrot, peeled and chopped
½ tsp dried tarragon
300 ml (½ pint) good homemade stock
400 g (14 oz) can haricot beans, drained (or cooked dried haricots – see pages 119–20)

Put the chicken, celery, tomatoes, onion, carrot, tarragon and stock in a casserole dish. Cover with a tight-fitting lid and cook in a moderate oven for 1 hour or until the chicken is tender and the vegetables are cooked. Stir in the beans and continue cooking for a further 15 minutes. Serve with mashed potato. Mash or liquidize the baby's portion as required.

Family meat loaf
750 g (1½ lb) very lean, finely minced beef
175 ml (6 fl oz) pure tomato juice
75 g (3 oz) porridge oats
2 large egg yolks
1 small onion, peeled and very finely chopped
1 tsp dried basil

Combine all the ingredients in a bowl then press into a 1 kg (2 lb) loaf tin. Bake in a moderate oven for 1–1½ hours. Serve with vegetables and tomato sauce. For a quick tomato sauce simmer 1 can chopped tomatoes with 1 tsp dried mixed herbs until thick. Mash or process the baby's portion as required and moisten with a little boiled water for freezing. Can be eaten cold with salads.

Fish with rice
500 g (1 lb) white filleted fish, steamed
250 g (8 oz) brown rice, cooked in unsalted boiling water for 30 minutes then drained
2 large eggs, hardboiled and chopped
4 tbsps cooked peas
2 tbsps chopped parsley
pinch of ground nutmeg
a little milk
3 tbsps natural yoghurt

Flake the fish, removing all bones, and combine with the rice, eggs, peas, parsley and nutmeg. Moisten with milk and add the natural yoghurt. Remove the baby's portion and mash or liquidize as required. Reheat when necessary. Do not add egg white for babies under eight months. For the rest of the family, put the fish and rice mixture into a buttered ovenproof dish. Cover with foil and heat through in a moderate oven for about 30–35 minutes. Serve with grilled tomatoes or salad.

Macaroni and fish bake (suitable for babies from six to eight months)
750 g (1½ lb) white fish fillets
approx. 600 ml (1 pint) milk
75 g (3 oz) macaroni
50 g (2 oz) margarine
40 g (1½ oz) plain flour
250 g (8 oz) frozen mixed vegetables
crushed cornflakes mixed with grated cheese for topping

Put the fish into a pan and barely cover with some of the milk. Cook gently for 15 to 20 minutes or until the fish flakes easily. Drain, reserving the cooking liquid, then remove any skin and bones from the fish and flake the flesh. Cook the macaroni according to the directions on the packet and drain. Make up the fish liquor to 600 ml (1 pint) with the remaining milk and place in a pan with the margarine and flour. Bring to the boil whisking continuously. Add the flaked fish, cooked macaroni and frozen mixed vegetables. Turn into a buttered ovenproof dish. When required, top with crushed cornflakes mixed with grated cheese and bake in a hot oven for 30–40 minutes.

Mediterranean fish casserole (suitable for babies over eight months)
4 thick fillets or steaks white fish, skinned
1 tbsp lemon juice
400 g (14 oz) can tomatoes
1 onion, peeled and chopped
1 level tsp dried basil
2 tbsps chopped parsley
125 g (4 oz) button mushrooms, washed

1 small green pepper, deseeded and chopped
50 g (2 oz) brown breadcrumbs
75 g (3 oz) cheese, grated

Put the fish into a well-buttered casserole dish and sprinkle with the lemon juice. Put the tomatoes, onion, basil and parsley in a pan and simmer for 10 minutes, then add the mushrooms and green pepper. Pour the sauce over the fish and bake, covered, in a moderate oven for 35 minutes. Combine the breadcrumbs and grated cheese and sprinkle over the casserole, then return to the oven for 15 minutes. Mash the baby's portion if required – it can be reheated if necessary. Serve with jacket potatoes or rice and a sprinkling of garlic salt for the adults.

VEGETARIAN CHOICES

Rice and vegetables Aurore
300–375 g (10–12 oz) brown rice
500 g (1 lb) packet frozen stir-fry vegetables
2 tbsps oil
Sauce:
600 ml (1 pint) milk
50 g (2 oz) plain flour
50 g (2 oz) margarine
3 tbsps tomato purée
50 g (2 oz) cheese, grated

Cook the rice in boiling water for 35 minutes, drain, cover and keep warm. Stir fry the vegetables in the oil and stir into the rice. Turn out on to a serving dish and keep warm. Put the milk, flour and margarine into a pan and bring to the boil, whisking continuously. Add the tomato purée and heat through without boiling. Pour the sauce over the rice and vegetables and sprinkle with the cheese, then brown under a hot grill. Mash or purée the baby's portion to a suitable consistency. If you have time use seasonal, fresh vegetables instead of frozen ones to make this dish.

Eggs Florentine (suitable for babies over nine months)
750 g (1½ lb) fresh spinach
25 g (1 oz) margarine
6 hardboiled eggs
450–600 ml (¾–1 pint) thick cheese sauce (see previous recipe)
75 g (3 oz) cheese, grated

Wash and drain the spinach. Place in a saucepan without any extra water, cover and cook over a low heat for 10–12 minutes, shaking the pan now and then. Drain and press out the excess water. Place in a serving dish and dot with the margarine. Halve the eggs and arrange on the spinach. Pour over the cheese sauce, sprinkle with the grated cheese and grill for 5 minutes until hot and bubbly. Eat with wholemeal bread.

Savoury nut stuffing
2 tbsps vegetable oil
1 onion, peeled and chopped
3 tomatoes, skinned, deseeded and chopped
250 g (8 oz) chopped nuts
4 Weetabix, crumbled
1 carrot, peeled and grated
300 ml (½ pint) vegetable stock (made by boiling vegetables such as carrots, celery, onion, cabbage and so on) with 1 tsp yeast extract added
1 tsp dried basil
1 egg, beaten

Heat the oil, gently fry the onion in it until softened, then add the tomatoes. Cook for a minute for two. Combine the nuts and Weetabix in a bowl then add the carrot, stock, basil, cooked onion and tomato. Add the egg to bind. Use this mixture to stuff marrow, courgettes, beefsteak tomatoes, even hollowed-out, peeled potatoes (cook in the oven with a little stock). It is also good made into 'sausage rolls', or formed into cakes, dipped in egg and breadcrumbs and fried until golden brown to make rissoles. Alternatively simply put the stuffing into a greased basin, steam for 1 hour and serve hot with tomato sauce and cooked vegetables.

Lentil burgers

250 g (8 oz) split red lentils, washed
300 ml (½ pint) water or homemade vegetable stock
1 bay leaf
1 large onion, peeled and finely chopped
1 tbsp chopped parsley
1 tbsp lemon juice
1 egg, beaten
50–75 g (2–3 oz) wholewheat breadcrumbs
oil for frying

Gently simmer the lentils, water or stock and bay leaf together in a non-stick pan for 25 minutes or until the lentils are tender. Remove the bay leaf, add the onion, parsley, lemon juice and egg and beat to a smooth, thick consistency. Cool the mixture slightly and shape into burgers. Coat each burger in the breadcrumbs, pressing firmly. Fry on both sides until crisp and golden and serve immediately.

To freeze: coat the burgers with breadcrumbs but do not cook them. Open-freeze then pack into a polythene bag when solid.

Sweetcorn bake

325 g (11 oz) can sweetcorn kernels
300 ml (½ pint) milk
2 eggs
50 g (2 oz) butter or margarine
150 g (5 oz) cheese, grated
2 medium parboiled potatoes, diced
50 g (2 oz) wholewheat breadcrumbs

Combine the corn and milk in a pan and slowly bring to the boil. Beat the eggs with a drop of the milk as it warms and stir into the hot milk and corn once it has come to the boil. Remove from the heat and add the butter or margarine, 125 g (4 oz) of the cheese, and the diced potatoes. Turn out into a greased ovenproof dish and cover with a mixture of the remaining grated cheese and the breadcrumbs. Bake in a moderate oven for 1 hour or until the topping is golden. Serve hot with grilled tomatoes and a green vegetable. Purée or mash your baby's portion.

Vegetarian casserole
625–750 g (1¼–1½ lb) mixed vegetables (see below)
3 tbsps oil
1 large onion, peeled and sliced
2 cloves garlic, crushed
2 tbsps plain flour
2 tbsps tomato purée
300 ml (½ pint) vegetable stock
1 bouquet garni
375 g (12 oz) potatoes, peeled and grated
125 g (4 oz) cheese, grated
1½ tbsps chopped parsley

Use whatever vegetables are available that you know your baby will
tolerate – leeks, carrots, cabbage, aubergine, courgettes, cooked beans,
swede or turnip, green pepper, celery and cauliflower are all suitable.
Cut them into chunks and put them in a casserole. Heat the oil and fry
the onion and garlic until golden. Stir in the flour, tomato purée,
stock, bay leaves and bouquet garni. Cook, stirring, for a minute or two
and then pour over the vegetables and set aside. Parboil the grated
potato for 3 minutes in boiling water, then drain and plunge into cold
water. Drain well, pressing out the water, then fluff with a fork and add
the grated cheese and chopped parsley. Spoon this mixture over the
vegetables and bake in a moderate oven for about 1½ hours. Before
serving brown under a hot grill. Mince or sieve a portion for your baby.
Unsuitable for freezing.

Cheese pudding
125 g (4 oz) wholewheat breadcrumbs
125 g (4 oz) cheese, grated
½ tsp mixed dried herbs
4 large eggs yolks, or 3 whole eggs if your baby is over eight months
450 ml (¾ pint) milk
a little margarine

Combine the breadcrumbs, cheese, herbs and eggs. Bring the milk to
the boil and pour over the cheese mixture. Mix well and pour into a
greased ovenproof dish. Dot with a little margarine and bake in a
moderate oven for 30–40 minutes until risen and brown. Serve with

baked beans – look for the additive-free, reduced-sugar variety.
Unsuitable for freezing.

Cheesy pasta
1 tbsp oil
375 g (12 oz) pasta shapes
175 g (6 oz) Mozzarella cheese, cut into cubes or grated

Bring a large saucepan of water to the boil and add the oil. Add the
pasta all at once and stir, then boil uncovered until tender – it should
be *al dente*, i.e. firm, but neither hard nor soggy. Fresh pasta cooks
much faster than dried pasta. Drain in a colander and stir in the cheese.
Serve with salad. Ideal finger food for an older baby.

Vegetarian hotpot*
250 g (8 oz) split red lentils
250 g (8 oz) long grain rice
4 small carrots, peeled and sliced
4 small sticks celery, diced
small piece of swede or turnip, chopped
1 can tinned tomatoes plus 2 tbsps juice
pinch of mixed dried herbs
chopped fresh parsley

Place all the ingredients except the parsley in a small saucepan and
barely cover with water. Gently simmer for 25 minutes, adding just
enough water to keep the stew from sticking to the bottom of the pan.
Drain and reserve the cooking juices. Purée or mash the stew with a
little chopped parsley and enough cooking liquid to give the required
consistency. Purée or mash according to your baby's stage of progress.
Suitable for freezing but only in puréed form. As your baby gets older
add a little chopped onion and yeast extract for a stronger flavour.

Eastern delight* (suitable for babies over eight months)
250 g (8 oz) dried haricot beans
3 tbsps cooking oil
1 large leek, washed and sliced
1 large red pepper, deseeded and chopped
2 carrots, peeled and chopped

2 sticks celery, chopped
75 g (3 oz) button mushrooms, wiped and sliced
400 g (14 oz) can tomatoes
1 tbsp tomato purée
1 tsp dried basil
2 tsp yeast extract dissolved in 600 ml (1 pint) cooking liquid from the
   beans
75 g (3 oz) bulgur wheat (available from health food shops)

Soak the beans overnight, rinse and place in a pan, covering with fresh
water. Bring to the boil and simmer for about 1 hour or until tender.
Drain, reserving the liquid for stock. In a flameproof casserole dish,
heat the oil and sauté the leek, red pepper, carrots, celery and
mushrooms for 5 minutes. Add the tomatoes, tomato purée, basil, and
yeast extract dissolved in cooking liquid. Cook for 10–15 minutes then
stir in the beans and bulgur wheat. Cover with a tight-fitting lid and
cook in a moderately hot oven for 45 minutes, adding more liquid if
necessary. Serve with bread.

Carrot and orange purée*
Scrub and slice 750 g (1½ lb) carrots and cook until just tender. Purée
with the juice of 1 large orange, return to the pan and heat through.
Use as an accompaniment to a main course. For adults and older
children stir a knob of butter or margarine into the purée to give a
glossy finish.

Parsnip, potato and apple purée*
Cook 750 g (1½ lb) peeled and chopped parsnips and 500 g (1 lb)
peeled and chopped potatoes until just tender. Cook 1 peeled, cored
and chopped dessert apple in 1 tbsp water until soft. Purée the
vegetables and apple together, return to a pan and heat through.
Remove the baby's portion. For the rest of the family, add ½ tsp ground
coriander and a knob of margarine. Heat gently for a few minutes then
serve.

Winter potage*
2 tbsps corn oil
1 medium onion, peeled and chopped
1 large carrot, scrubbed and sliced

1 small parsnip, peeled and sliced
1 small turnip, peeled and chopped
1 medium potato, peeled and sliced
1 chunk swede, peeled and chopped
1 stick celery, chopped
600 ml (1 pint) water
2 tbsps tomato purée
1 tsp mixed dried herbs
seasoning
chopped parsley to garnish

Heat the oil and fry the onion for 3 minutes. Add the rest of the
vegetables, the water, tomato purée, herbs and a little seasoning. Stir
well, bring to the boil and simmer for 25–30 minutes, adding more
liquid if necessary. Liquidize the soup, or part-liquidize if you prefer a
chunky texture, and reheat. Serve garnished with the chopped parsley.
If it seems to be too runny for your baby, mash in a little cooked potato
to thicken.

Shepherdess pie
250 g (8 oz) split red lentils
250 g (8 oz) turnips, peeled and chopped
250 g (8 oz) parsnips, peeled and chopped
1 carrot, scrubbed and sliced
1 bay leaf
250 g (8 oz) swede, peeled and chopped
500 g (1 lb) potatoes, peeled and chopped
knob of margarine
a little milk
125 g (4 oz) cheese, grated

Put the lentils into a pan with the turnips, parsnips, carrot and bay leaf.
Add just enough water to stop the vegetables sticking to the pan and
simmer for 20–25 minutes until the vegetables are tender. Drain if
necessary. Remove the bay leaf and turn out into a 1.5 l (2½ pint)
ovenproof dish. Simmer the swede and potatoes together until tender,
drain, then mash with a knob of margarine and a drop of milk. Spread
over the lentil mixture and mark the surface with a fork. Sprinkle with
the grated cheese and bake in a moderate oven for 20–25 minutes.

Serve with a green salad. As your baby gets older add a little yeast
extract to the lentil mixture for extra flavour.

Mixed root vegetable gratin (suitable for babies over eight months)
750 g (1½ lb) mixed root vegetables, peeled and chopped
125 g (4 oz) cheese, grated
2 large eggs, beaten
3 tbsps natural yoghurt
seasoning
50 g (2 oz) wholewheat breadcrumbs

Simmer the root vegetables until tender then drain and mash with the
grated cheese. Stir in the eggs and yoghurt then season lightly. Pile into
an ovenproof dish and fork over the surface. Sprinkle with the
wholewheat breadcrumbs and bake in a hot oven for about 30 minutes.
Delicious on its own or as an accompaniment.

Baby nut roast
This could be given to your baby when the family is having a more
sophisticated nut roast.

2 tbsps wholewheat breadcrumbs
2 tbsps unsalted ground nuts
1 tin tomatoes mashed
1 egg yolk or, for babies over 8 months, ½ beaten egg
pinch dried mixed herbs or 1 tsp chopped parsley
¼ small, very finely chopped onion (for babies over 7 months)
knob of margarine

Moisten the breadcrumbs with a drop of boiling water then add all the
remaining ingredients except the margarine. Mix well and spoon into a
small, greased ovenproof dish. Dot with the margarine, cover with foil
and bake for 20–25 minutes in a moderate oven. For a change add a
little grated mild cheese.

Cheesy carrot and celeriac
250 g (8 oz) carrots, peeled and sliced
250 g (8 oz) celeriac, peeled and sliced
1 tbsp lemon juice

175 g (6 oz) low-fat cream cheese
½ tsp mixed dried herbs or 1 tsp fresh herbs

Put the carrots, celeriac and lemon juice into a pan, barely cover with
water and simmer until the vegetables are tender – about 20 minutes.
Drain and return to the pan. Beat the cream cheese and herbs together
and add to the pan. Stir over a gentle heat until the cheese has coated
the vegetables then serve with salad and wholemeal bread. Sieve or
mash the baby's portion.

PUDDINGS

Apricot almond semolina
750 ml (1¼ pints) milk
65 g (2½ oz) semolina
2 tbsps sugar
50 g (2 oz) ground almonds
1 small tin apricots in natural juice, drained and chopped

Bring the milk to the boil and sprinkle over the semolina. Whisk over a
gentle heat for 2 to 3 minutes. Remove from the heat and stir in the
sugar and ground almonds. Serve immediately, decorated with the
chopped apricots. Reheat the baby's portion as required, mashing the
apricots into the semolina first.

Baked tapioca pudding
900 ml (1½ pints) milk
65 g (2½ oz) tapioca
2 tbsps soft brown sugar
½ tsp ground cinnamon
25 g (1 oz) sultanas
3 dessert apples cored, peeled and sliced
1 tsp natural vanilla essence
50 g (2 oz) ground almonds

Bring the milk to the boil, add the tapioca and simmer for 10 minutes.
Remove from the heat and add the rest of the ingredients. Pour into a
buttered ovenproof dish and bake in a low oven for about 1 hour.
Liquidize the baby's portion if required.

Homemade yoghurt
Take 600 ml (1 pint) ordinary milk to which has been added 1 tbsp
dried milk powder. Heat to boiling point to kill any bacteria. Remove
from the heat, cover and leave to cool until just comfortably warm.
Add 1 tbsp natural yoghurt as a starter and whisk well. Pour into a
wide-necked Thermos flask and seal. Leave undisturbed for six hours.
Turn the yoghurt into a clean, airtight container and stir – it may be
quite thin at this stage but thickens when chilled. Seal and store in the
refrigerator. Reserve a little of each batch of yoghurt to begin the next.
Begin with new yoghurt after a couple of months. It is a good idea to
keep a flask solely for making yoghurt and keep it filled with water with
a few drops of sterilizing solution added.

Apricot glories
250 g (8 oz) dried apricots
water and orange juice to cover
2–3 tbsps ground almonds
natural yoghurt
clear honey (optional)

Wash the apricots, put into a medium-sized saucepan and just cover
with water and orange juice. Leave to soak for a couple of hours then
simmer for 30 minutes or until soft and syrupy. Cool and stir in the
ground almonds. Liquidize until smooth, adding a drop of orange juice
if too thick. Layer the apricot purée with the natural yoghurt in glasses.
If you need to, sweeten the yoghurt first with a little clear honey. You
can decorate this with toasted flaked almonds for the rest of the family.

Apple jelly dessert
Dissolve a lemon jelly in 150 ml (¼ pint) unsweetened apple purée and
stir in 2 tbsps sultanas. Make up to 450 ml (¾ pint) with warm boiled
water. Leave to cool then chill until set. Decorate with ratafia biscuits
and whipped cream for the adults.

Apple ice (suitable for babies over eight months)
Whip 300 ml (½ pint) whipping cream until it stands in peaks. Add
300 ml (½ pint) unsweetened apple purée. Turn out into a shallow
container and freeze until firm.

Custard ice-cream (suitable for babies over eight months)
4 large eggs, beaten
600 ml (1 pint) single cream
50 g (2 oz) sugar
2 tbsps natural vanilla essence

Put the eggs, cream and sugar into a basin over a pan of gently
simmering water. Cook, stirring all the time, until the custard coats the
back of a wooden spoon. Add the vanilla essence and cool. Pour into a
container and fast freeze, stirring now and then.
Brown bread ice-cream: make up the custard as above. Cool, then stir in
the vanilla essence and add 65 g (2½ oz) brown breadcrumbs which
have been previously fried in butter and then cooled. Freeze as above.

Banana dream*
2 small dessert apples, peeled and cored
1 small, ripe banana
1 tsp lemon juice
1 level tbsp ground almonds
1 tsp sugar

Process the apples in a food processor until coarsely chopped, or chop it
by hand. Add the banana, lemon juice, ground almonds and honey.
Purée. Leftovers are nice as a spread on French bread for the rest of the
family.

Quick banana ice-cream
Whisk 400 g (14 oz) can chilled evaporated milk until thick and whisk
in 75 g (3 oz) soft brown sugar. Mash 3 bananas with 1 tbsp lemon
juice. Whisk into the evaporated milk. Spoon into a large plastic
container and freeze until firm.

Bread and butter pudding (suitable for babies over eight months)
8 slices wholemeal bread, minus crusts, spread thinly with margarine or
    butter
125 og (4 oz) currants and/or sultanas
grated rind of 1 lemon
75 g (3 oz) soft brown sugar
nutmeg

3 eggs
600 ml (1 pint) milk

Grease a fairly large ovenproof dish. Cut the bread into squares and
layer it in the dish with the dried fruit, lemon rind and sugar, ending
with a layer of bread, buttered side uppermost. Sprinkle with sugar and
ground nutmeg. Beat the eggs and add to the milk. Pour over the
pudding and leave to soak for 30 minutes. Cook in a moderate oven for
1 hour or until golden. Serve with custard if you like.

Rice pudding
65 g (2½ oz) carolina or pudding rice
25 g (1 oz) sugar
600 ml (1 pint) milk
nutmeg
margarine

Put the rice, sugar and milk into a greased ovenproof dish. Sprinkle
with the ground nutmeg and dot with margarine. Bake in a moderate
oven for 20 minutes, stir well, then continue cooking on a low heat for
1 to 1½ hours or until the rice is tender. Serve hot with stewed fruit or
cold with chopped fresh fruit.

Apple Charlotte*
50 g (2 oz) polyunsaturated margarine
500 g (1 lb) cooking apples, peeled, cored and sliced
125 g (4 oz) wholewheat breadcrumbs
75 g (3 oz) soft brown sugar
grated rind of 1 lemon
2 tbsps water

Grease a medium pie dish with some of the margarine. Add layers of
apples, breadcrumbs, sugar, lemon rind and dots of margarine, ending
with a layer of breadcrumbs. Pour over the water and dot with
margarine. Bake in a moderate oven for 45 minutes to 1 hour. Serve
with custard or natural yoghurt.

Blackcurrant jelly
Dissolve 15 g (½ oz) sachet powdered gelatine in 4 tbsps hot water. Stir

in undiluted pure blackcurrant juice to make up to 600 ml (1 pint) and chill until set. Some babies dislike chilled food; if this applies to your baby, serve at room temperature.

Fluffy milk jelly (suitable for babies over eight months)
3 eggs, separated
600 ml (1 pint) whole milk
25 g (1 oz) sugar
few drops natural vanilla essence
15 g (½ oz) powdered gelatine

Mix together the egg yolks, milk, sugar and vanilla. Dissolve the gelatine in 4 tbsps hot water and slowly whisk into the milk mixture. Chill until nearly set. Whisk the egg whites until stiff and fold into the jelly. Pour into a serving dish and chill until set. Serve plain or with fruit.

TEATIME TREATS

As your child grows older you will be able to increase her range of food. Here are some toddler favourites.

Celery dip
Mix 250 g (8 oz) fromage frais or fromage blanc with 3 sticks finely chopped celery. Chill. Serve with raw vegetable pieces, such as cauliflower, carrot and cucumber, for dipping. You can also dip crisps, rusks, biscuits in it. You can make this dip using sieved cottage cheese and natural yoghurt.

Crunchy spiced chicken
This teatime treat will go down better than the fast-food store variety and is healthier.
Allow 1 boneless chicken breast per person. Dip in beaten egg then in wholemeal breadcrumbs flavoured with a little paprika, grated Parmesan cheese and mixed dried herbs. Place on a greased baking tray and bake in a moderate oven, turning once, until crisp and golden. This will take 30–45 minutes depending on size. Serve hot with jacket potatoes topped with natural yoghurt or low-fat cream cheese.

Perfect pizza
125 g (4 oz) wholemeal flour
125 g (4 oz) self-raising flour
1 tbsp wheatgerm
pinch of salt
1 tsp baking powder
1 tsp dried mixed herbs
50 g (2 oz) polyunsaturated margarine
1 egg, beaten
milk to mix
ingredients for topping (see below)

For the base, combine the wholemeal flour, self-raising flour, wheatgerm, salt, baking powder and herbs. Rub in the polyunsaturated margarine. Add the egg and enough milk to form a soft dough, mixing gently. Wrap in cling film and chill before using. Roll the dough out to a 20–22.5 cm (8–9 inch) circle and place on a greased baking tray. Top with anything your toddler likes. Choose from flaked tuna fish, chopped ham, sliced mushrooms, chopped red and green peppers, sliced tomatoes, sweetcorn kernels etc. Finish off with lots of grated cheese and bake in a hot oven for 30 minutes. Serve hot or cold with a side salad.

Beefburger (another alternative to junk food varieties)
750 g (1½ lb) minced beef
1 medium onion, finely chopped
1 tbsp finely chopped fresh parsley
2 tbsps breadcrumbs
2 tbsps wheatgerm
seasoning
natural yoghurt to bind

Combine the minced beef, onion, parsley, breadcrumbs and wheatgerm and mix well. Lightly season and bind together with a little natural yoghurt. Divide into 8 equal portions and form into flat cakes, pressing firmly. Cover and chill for several hours before cooking. Grill on high for 8 minutes, turning once. The burgers should be dark brown on both sides and a skewer inserted into the centre should produce colourless juices. Serve with wholemeal baps and a salad garnish.

Nut spread (excellent on sandwiches for finger feeding)
Beat 2 tablespoons ground unsalted nuts into 1 small carton low-fat
cream cheese and flavour with a drop of fruit juice or some chopped
parsley. Spread on wholemeal bread.

Family vegetable soup
750 g (1½ lb) chopped mixed vegetables, such as potato, onion, carrot,
  celery, swede, cabbage, leek, cauliflower, parsnip
50 g (2 oz) butter
1.2 l (2 pints) stock
2 tbsps tomato purée
2 tsps dried mixed herbs

Fry the vegetables in the butter for 5 minutes then add the stock,
tomato purée and herbs. Simmer for about 30 minutes, adding more
liquid if necessary. Liquidize briefly and reheat. As a variation, add
some small pasta shapes before reheating and cook for 10 minutes.

Pasta salad
50 g (2 oz) red kidney beans, soaked overnight then drained
75 g (3 oz) pasta shapes, cooked, rinsed and drained
75 g (3 oz) Cheddar cheese, diced
50 g (2oz) cooked peas
1 stick celery, cleaned and chopped
1 tbsp lemon juice
1 tbsp chopped parsley
natural yoghurt to bind or serve separately
lettuce leaves
1 large tomato, sliced

Place the red kidney beans in fresh water, bring to the boil, boil hard
for 15 minutes then reduce the heat and simmer until tender. Drain
and cool. Mix with the cooked pasta, Cheddar, peas, celery, lemon
juice and parsley. Stir in the yoghurt or serve separately. Chill then
serve on a bed of lettuce garnished with the sliced tomato.

Pasta salads are great favourites with toddlers. Ring the changes with
tuna fish, chopped hardboiled egg, chopped ham, cooked french beans,
sweetcorn and so on.

Egg on a bed
Spread a toasted crumpet with yeast extract and top with a poached egg.

Eggy bread
Beat 2 eggs together with 1 tbsp milk. Soak 4 slices wholewheat bread in this mixture. Fry in a little oil in a non-stick frying pan. This can either be served as a savoury, or with a squeeze of orange juice and a dribble of honey as a sweet.

Peanut fingers
Spread wholewheat toast with peanut butter. Top with grated cheese and grill. Serve cut into fingers.

Pizza toasts
Use large, thick slices of wholemeal bread and toast one side only. Spread the untoasted sides with a little tomato purée. Arrange some fried bacon, mashed sardines or tuna on the bread, and add thin rings of red or green pepper. Top with thick slices of Cheddar cheese, and a slice of fresh tomato. Grill until hot and bubbly. Serve with salad or baked beans.

Fishy potatoes
4 large baking potatoes
1 large tin tuna, drained and flaked
2 tbsps chopped parsley
2 eggs

Scrub the potatoes, prick them with a fork and bake them in a hot oven for 1¼ hours or until tender. Cut the potatoes in half lengthways, and scoop out the insides. Mash with the tuna, parsley and eggs. Cover and chill until required. Bake in a hot oven for 25–30 minutes until golden. Serve with salad.

Cheesy bacon puffs
250 g (8 oz) chopped fried bacon
3 tbsps mango or peach chutney
150 g (5 oz) Cheddar cheese, grated
1 medium onion, peeled and finely chopped

400 g (14 oz) packet frozen puff pastry, thawed
a little beaten egg

Combine the bacon, chutney, cheese and onion. Roll out the pastry to
a 40 × 30 cm (16 × 12 inch) rectangle and cut into 8 squares. Divide
the filling between the squares. Dampen edges and fold over into
triangles, pressing firmly. Place on a baking sheet, cover and chill until
required. Brush with beaten egg and bake for 25–30 minutes in a hot
oven. Serve hot with baked beans or grilled tomatoes, or cold with
salad.

Spanish-style omelette
3 tbsps corn oil
1 onion, peeled and chopped
125 g (4 oz) leftover cooked potato, diced
250 g (8 oz) frozen mixed vegetables, heated through and drained
7 large eggs
good handful chopped parsley
seasoning

Heat the oil in a medium-sized non-stick pan and fry the onion until
softened. Add the potato and mixed vegetables. Beat the eggs with the
parsley and season to taste. Pour the eggs into the pan and cook. When
the underside is brown, transfer the pan to under the grill and cook
until the top is set and golden. Cut into wedges and serve immediately
with wholemeal bread and grilled tomatoes.

Cheese soufflé rarebits
Use medium-thick slices of wholemeal bread and allow 1 large egg per
slice. Toast the bread on one side and spread the untoasted side with a
little tomato purée. Top with cooked sliced ham and slices of cheese.
Separate the eggs and beat the yolks with a tiny drop of milk. Whisk up
the egg whites stiffly and fold into the yolks. Spoon on to the toasts and
bake in a moderate oven for 15–20 minutes. Serve with salad.

Potato salad
Combine diced, cooked potato with a little chopped fresh parsley and
moisten with natural yoghurt. Sprinkle with diced hardboiled egg and
crushed, crisply fried bacon.

Tuna dip

Blend a small can of tuna fish, drained, with enough natural yoghurt to make a sauce, then add a dash of lemon juice and a little chopped fresh parsley. Serve your baby's portion in an egg cup on a plate with tiny sticks of celery, carrot and cucumber and sprigs of cauliflower.

INDEX

Additives, 29, 89–93, 106
Afterpains, 6
Allergies, 2, 15, 23, 29, 78, 83–93
  prevention of, 93
Amino acids, 57, 78
Anaemia, 60
Antioxidants, 85
Apple Charlotte recipe, 125
Apple ice recipe, 123
Apple jelly dessert recipe, 123
Apricot almond semolina recipe, 122
Apricot glories recipe, 123
Aspartame, 86
Asthma, 92

Baked tapioca pudding recipe, 122
Balanced diet, 40, 46–8
Bananas
  banana dream, 124
  quick banana ice-cream, 124
Beefburger recipe, 127
Blackcurrant jelly recipe, 125
Body shape, 70
Bottle-feeding, 13–21
  changing from breast, 20
  choice of formula, 14–15
  frequency of feeds, 15, 19
  last bottle, 21
  making up bottles, 15–16
  reasons for, 14
  sterilizing bottles, 18–19
  warming up bottles, 16–17
Bras, 4
Bread and butter pudding recipe, 124
Breast-feeding, 1–13
  changing to bottle, 20
  enjoyment of, 3
  frequency of feeds, 10
  organizations, 13
  positioning for, 9, 10
  and premature babies, 94–5

  in public, 12
  reasons for, 2
  tips, 8
  underfeeding, 10
  and work, 12–13
Breast milk, 1, 6–9
  appearance of, 7
  expressed, 12, 94–5
Breast pumps, 94–5

Calcium, 59, 81
Calories, 58, 69–71
Carbohydrates, 56–7
Carrot and orange purée recipe, 119
Cassettes for soothing baby, 11–12
Cauliflower cheese recipe, 108
Celery dip recipe, 126
Centile charts, 65–6, 72
Cheese, 26
  cauliflower cheese recipe, 108
  cheese soufflé rarebits recipe, 130
  cheesy bacon puffs recipe, 129
  cheesy carrot and celeriac recipe, 121
  cheesy pasta recipe, 118
  pudding recipe, 117
Chicken
  casserole recipe, 107
  chicken and bean pot recipe, 111
  crunchy spiced chicken recipe, 126
  roast chicken recipe, 111
Cholesterol, 55
Coeliac disease, 73, 98–100
Colic, 88, 90
Colostrum, 5, 6–7
Combining foods, 45, 57, 78
Commercial baby food, 28–30
Complementary bottles, 8, 11
Conflicts over food, 40, 49–51
Constipation, 20
Cow's milk, unmodified, 27–8, 42, 53–4, 59, 90

Mother & Baby

MAGAZINE

your pregnancy and childcare expert

With a baby on the way, it is important to keep track of the latest developments on all aspects of motherhood, from conception through to the early years with your new baby.

Mother & Baby magazine is Britain's best monthly guide, packed with exclusive reports and lively features for you and your growing family.

Regular sections on pregnancy and birth, your baby and toddler, family relationships and health and medicine offer factual information and expert advice which will continue to support you throughout the coming months and years . . . Plus a special colour section on the lighter side of motherhood, with fashion tips for you and your child, things to make and do, and lots of free gifts and special offers in every issue.

So make sure you don't miss a single issue of **Mother & Baby**. Have the next 12 issues delivered straight to your door, postage free, for only £12.00 – plus a full money-back guarantee if you decide to cancel at any time!

Simply call our *Subscription Hotline* direct on 0235 865656 with details of your Access or Visa card, and we'll take care of the rest. Or, if you prefer, complete the coupon below and post the whole page to:

Mother & Baby, FREEPOST, PO Box 35, Abingdon, Oxon OX14 3BR.
